Acclaim for
Muscle Boys: Gay Gym Culture

"Alvarez clearly knows his territory."

—*The Gay & Lesbian Review*

"Accessible prose and experienced insight. This book provides the reader with a timely idea: the importance of the gym in allowing gay men a place where they can find each other and, most significantly, themselves. This very readable book politely kicks sand in the faces of those who impugn the gym as anything other than a unique, healthy, surprisingly diverse communal culture worthy of study, comment, and maybe even membership. This insightful history gives voice to the countless gay men who found the strength to assert themselves and in doing so redefined masculinity."

—Tom Cardamone,
Author, *The Werewolves of Central Park*

"An informed history and breezy analysis of gay men's thirsty interest in body image. Athlete Alvarez is a trainer who leaves his muscular signature on this entertaining book that covers early physique magazines, steroids, and pro athletes like Dave Kopay and Tom Waddell, inventor of the Gay Games. As a longtime gym-insider, Alvarez writes about what he knows. He captures the mystery and history of gay gym culture, of self-fashioning notions of masculine identity, and how gay muscle flexed gay power and uncloseted our Platonic Ideals into straight mainstream advertising."

—Jack Fritscher, PhD,
Author, "Gay Sports" in *Gay San Francisco: Eyewitness Drummer — Sex, Art, and the Salon Around* Drummer Magazine

Muscle Boys
Gay Gym Culture

Muscle Boys
Gay Gym Culture

Erick Alvarez

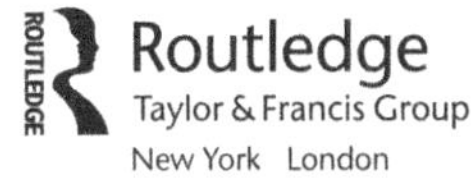

First published by

The Haworth Press, Taylor & Francis Group, 270 Madison Ave., New York, NY 10016.

This edition published 2012 by Routledge
711 Third Avenue, New York, NY 10017
2 Park Square, Milton Park, Abingdon, Oxon OX14 4RN

PUBLISHER'S NOTES
The development, preparation, and publication of this work has been undertaken with great care. However, the Publisher, employees, editors, and agents of The Haworth Press are not responsible for any errors contained herein or for consequences that may ensue from use of materials or information contained in this work. The Haworth Press is committed to the dissemination of ideas and information according to the highest standards of intellectual freedom and the free exchange of ideas. Statements made and opinions expressed in this publication do not necessarily reflect the views of the Publisher, Directors, management, or staff of The Haworth Press, Inc., or an endorsement by them.

Identities and circumstances of individuals discussed in this book have, in some cases, been changed to protect confidentiality.

Cover design by Jennifer M. Gaska.

Library of Congress Cataloging-in-Publication Data

Alvarez, Erick.
Muscle boys : gay gym culture / Erick Alvarez.
p. cm.
Includes bibliographical references and index.
ISBN: 978-1-56023-404-3 (soft)
1. Gay culture. 2. Gay men—Social life and customs. 3. Body image in men. 4. Gymnasiums—Social aspects. 5. Physical fitness—Social aspects. 6. Body, Human-Social aspects. I. Title.

HQ76.96.A58 2007
306.76'62097309045—dc22

2007017273

Para Aracelly, mi adorada madre.

Gracias mamá por apoyarme en todos
mis proyectos y aventuras, aunque

algunos fuesen tan extraños y atrevidos como el escribir un libro.

ABOUT THE AUTHOR

Erick Alvarez, BS, grew up in San Francisco, where he attended San Francisco State University and earned his degree in kinesiology and exercise science. *Muscle Boys* is his first book. For more information, check out www.erickalvarez.com and www.gaygymculture.com.

CONTENTS

List of Figures

Muscle Boys: Gay Gym Culture
Published by The Haworth Press, Taylor & Francis Group, 2008.
doi:10.1300/6034_a

Acknowledgments

With much love and gratitude I thank John De Cecco for his ongoing support and for believing in me even when I had doubts. To have such an eminent scholar as my chief editor was more than I could have asked for. John is a true pioneer of the GLBT movement and of the field of human sexuality, and discussing at length our history and sexuality exceeded every expectation of my inquisitive mind. But most important, to be able to call him not just my mentor but also a close friend is an honor I will carry with me always.

I am deeply indebted to my writing mentor and independent editor, Mandy Erickson, for helping me transform my thoughts, questions, ideas, and research into this book. Without her friendship, support, and encouragement this book would not have been possible. Her unmatched patience and ferocious command of the craft are gifts that I can only aspire to.

You cannot tell the story of a group of people unless they share it with you. So, I owe a colossal thank-you to the almost 6,000 men who took the time to share with me their lives, stories, views, and opinions by participating in my interviews and surveys. To each and every one of you, I thank you.

Getting men to talk can be a difficult task, getting them to share their very private lives ever harder . . . so finding those who are willing is priceless. With that, a big kudos goes to Andy Wysocki and Bill Sanderson of bigmuscle.com and bigmusclebear.com for helping me reach the thousands of men from around the world who participated in my research.

Thank you, Robert Mainardi and Trent Dunphy of The Magazine Archives, Dennis Bell of Athletic Model Guild, and John Rutherford of Colt Studio, not only for providing me with such an amazing compilation of photographs but also for sharing with me your knowledge and expertise.

Muscle Boys: Gay Gym Culture
Published by The Haworth Press, Taylor & Francis Group, 2008.
doi:10.1300/6034_b

Chapter 1

Gay Gym Culture

This book started as a study of the gay gym, that cultural phenomenon and, until recently, somewhat obscure social institution that first surfaced during the 1970s in the gay ghettos of San Francisco, West Hollywood, and New York. But as I started consulting references and interviewing gay men at gay gyms, I had some important realizations: One, there is a startling number of gay men who are sharing a lifestyle; that it is them who make the gym gay; and, that over the past three decades, they have created a subculture all of their own. Two, in comparing one gay gym with another, even within the same city, the dynamics of one gay gym can be dramatically different from the others' depending on the demographics of each particular one (younger men, older men, bears, circuit boys, etc). Third, and most important, that far away from the gay ghettos, in every American city, suburb, and rural area, as well as abroad, gay men of every age, race, ethnicity, and socioeconomic status are living and practicing the lifestyle established by the gay gym and revolving around new norms in terms of aesthetics, body image, self-image, athletics, socialization, and, most important, interpersonal relationships. Because of these realizations, the book shifted its focus from the gym to the gay men who go to the gym and the social ethos that brings them together. These men are better described by the popular jargon used today: *muscle boys*.

In less than two decades, the physical and social trends of the gay gym have propagated far from the gay ghettos of San Francisco and New York; this is largely due to travel habits of modern gay men and the use of the Internet. The culture of the gay gym has been globalized. What had once been the domain of a small number of trendy gay men in urban enclaves is now a lifestyle for many gay men—urban, suburban, and rural. The gay gym has become a cultural trend, a sub-

Muscle Boys: Gay Gym Culture
Published by The Haworth Press, Taylor & Francis Group, 2008.
doi:10.1300/6034_01

culture all on its own. This subculture—*gay gym culture*—is what this book is about.

The body culture of the gay gym—identified by a focus on a built muscular body—is most present in media, but it has come to affect gay life in many ways, from the way we identify and describe ourselves to the way we meet for sex, dating, or more serious relationships. Simply browsing at the personal ads on any popular gay Web site is case in point that lifestyles built around working out and the gym are used not just to describe an increasing number of gay men, but desired and sometimes required from their potential partners and friends.

In the most basic socialization between gay men, the longstanding "What do you do?" has been replaced by "Where do you work out?" From mating to entertainment, gay gym culture has become such a powerful and influential ethos that unless you isolate yourself from gay life it affects you one way or another. Whether you are twenty-two or forty-nine, and whether you are a self-described gym rat or you have never set foot in a gym, if you are a gay or bisexual man living today, then this book is also about you.

In this chapter we will take a look at the demographic that makes up modern gay gym culture and discuss its stereotypes and ideals. We will look at Western history, dating back to the Greeks, to find out where gay gym culture came from, because in examining how a subculture emerged and evolved in the first place we get more than statistics—we begin to understand it. Last, I will discuss the most visible product of the gay gym—the gym-built body—and the role that it plays in modern gay society.

WHAT IS GAY GYM CULTURE?

Gay gym culture is somewhat confusing because the entire genre often gets categorized under one group as if it was made up entirely of an identical set of men. Yet my research shows that it is made up of a diverse group of men: the gym and issues associated with it can represent very different things. For this reason I have identified the six principal subgroups that make up gym culture today:

1. *The Muscle Boy*—This is the largest group within gay gym culture; it is made up of eighteen-year-olds to men in their forties who do not strongly identify with some of the other subcultures of the gym such as the circuit or bear culture.

2. *The Older Male*—The forty-plus group is largely made up by gay Baby Boomers, many of whom have been active at the gym for years and even decades. For this group, health is becoming the number-one reason for participation in the gym, with socialization and aesthetics coming in second and third.

3. *The Poz Jock*—This group is made up HIV-positive men who use the gym and exercise as an important aspect of managing HIV and AIDS. Bodybuilders by default, this group has been very influential in introducing steroids into gym culture and determining current standards of musculature and definition for the male body.

4. *The Athlete*—Sports men and jocks make up this group. For these men, the gym is an extension of their sport, a cross-training tool. This group is largely made up of noncompetitive, recreational athletes, and sometimes includes elite and professional athletes.

5. *The Circuit Boy*—Party boys and men make up this group. They train hard to meet the standards of the circuit and have the strength and endurance to party all weekend. A cosmetic athlete, the circuit boy is for the most part influenced by the high beauty standards and aesthetics of the circuit and gay urban nightlife.

6. *The Muscle Bear*—One of the newest additions and fastest-growing groups within gym culture. Big, burly, and strong as hell, these unconventional guys are not concerned with looking pretty. Real men, they say, look buff, hairy, and rugged.

Why It Matters

Gay gym culture is present in just about every aspect of gay media and gay life. Open up a magazine, watch any of the gay-themed television shows, or attend a gay social event, and the product of the gay gym—the gym-built body—is there to remind you.

Browse through the personals ads online or any gay newspaper or magazine and you will find only a few out of thousands that do not use the parameters and ideals of the gay gym to describe their body types. Interests based on particular body types, fitness-related lifestyles, and gym-related social activities, all associated with gym culture, often determine what it is that gay men today are looking for in a potential mate. In short, gay gym culture has become a very influential part of modern gay identity.

In this book I will candidly examine just how much the ideals set forth by the gay gym affect the many aspects of modern gay cultural life and in doing so discuss the following questions:

- Why do we go to the gym?
- How is the gym connected to modern gay socialization?
- How does gay gym culture influence self-esteem?
- How does body image affect sex, dating, and relationships?
- What is the connection between masculinity and muscles?
- Is the gay athlete a new phenomenon, or is he just out of the closet?
- How does the party scene and circuit culture shape our ideals about body image?
- What is the role of the gym in the aging process for older gay men?
- Why are gay men using steroids? How did the trend start?
- What is the role of the media and the porn star in our standards, fantasies, and ideals?
- Why does the locker room generate much controversy, anxiety, and excitement among gay men?

Gay gym culture carries a lot of weight (not just literally) because it is establishing a social structure and hierarchy, and gay men are increasingly using the parameters of gym culture to identify socially. Our identification within these groups comes quite close to the heart, affecting and—to a large extent—deciding our choices for friends, sex partners, dates, and even life partners. When it comes to socializing, the gym and our relationships to our bodies are equally as important—if not more so—as socio-economic status or education level.

Methods Used

I first surveyed and interviewed 200 gay and bisexual men in San Francisco at the various gay and gay-trafficked gyms. Respondents came in all shapes and sizes, races, ethnicities, and across the socioeconomic stratum. They were Asian, white, Latino, African American, and every mix in between. They came young and old, and included those with a high school education and those with PhDs.

Some identify as bears or athletes, others as circuit boys, some have been working out for thirty days and others for thirty years.

The demographics of the respondents were so diverse that I became interested in expanding my research outside of San Francisco. With the help of Andy Wysocki and Bill Sanderson, publishers of two of the most popular muscle-bound Web destinations in the world (bigmuscle.com and bigmusclebear.com), I conducted an online survey. Andy and Bill posted information about my research for this book with a link to the survey on both Web sites making it available to the combined 40,000 members (at the time) of bigmuscle.com and bigmusclebear.com. Members of both Web sites were given the option to take the survey anonymously; I explained in a disclaimer that their answers and information obtained would, in part or whole, be published in this book.*

The results were overwhelming. *Five thousand five hundred and seventy six* gay and bisexual men around the world took part in the survey. Respondents were as young as fifteen and as old as seventy-nine, and they came from as far north as Iceland and as far south as Argentina, and from as Westernized-as-it-gets Los Angeles and Dallas to cities such as Kuala Lumpur and Dubai—they hailed from a total of sixty-five different countries. Crawfish farmers and opera conductors alike shared their feelings, experiences, thoughts, and concerns about the issues this book discusses, from body image and steroids to sports and sex in the locker room.

In addition to the data that surveys and interviews can provide, my professional life for a period of twelve years took place at the center of gay gym culture. From 1992 to 2005, I worked as a personal trainer at gay gyms throughout San Francisco. During this period I closely worked with and trained hundreds of gay men, while meeting thousands more. Some of these interactions lasted a few minutes, and others a few years, and in the process I've come to learn and understand what gay gym culture is and what drives the muscle boys. I present to you over a decade of observation and thought, an intimate insider's account of what gay gym culture and muscle boys are all about.

---

*To ensure accuracy, the survey was conducted utilizing surveymonkey.com software. The survey was posted on bigmuscle.com and bigmusclebear.com. When a member took the survey, the member was directed to the surveymonkey.com Web site. Members of both Web sites have to be registered with valid e-mail addresses to avoid "bogus" takers.

STEREOTYPES

In each of the chapters in this book that covers a particular subgroup of gay men, I discuss the gym and the reasons that this distinct group involves itself with the gym. Although I will explain the general aspects of a given group and even though most of us have a tendency to attach a person to a group or to a stereotype, it should be made clear that because it is also in our nature to be multifaceted, many of us oscillate between groups and subcultures. However, because every group within gym culture has a stereotype attached to it, let's look at what this means.

Humans are social animals; as far back as we know we have lived and traveled in herds. It is our nature to gravitate toward groups of those that are like us, and, in the process, we get stereotyped as representative of that group. Stereotypes are more than a hypothetical representation of a set of rules and norms; they are the generalized version of these rules and norms. Stereotypes are largely a mental picture of what other people are like.

In the gay community, most of the subcultures seem to have a body type attached (i.e., jock, bear, muscle boy, leather man, circuit-boy, twink, etc.). It is interesting to ponder to what extent our body types determine the social circumstances we will end up in. How much does our physique open doors, and how much does it close them? An entire generation of young gay men is growing up and socializing based on how they are built and what they look like, and this will, no doubt, have a weighty effect on the future of gay culture. Avoiding stereotypes does not help us overcome them; understanding them does.

With this in mind, in this book we will discuss the muscle boy stereotypes and subcultures for what they are, not because they are good or bad. Yet in fully understanding them, we will also discuss the perceptions, negative and positive, associated with each. For this reason I invite you to also look at these subgroups as stages in a person's life. The muscle boy will be part of that group only as long as he is of a specific age, the circuit boy will be part of that group as long as his ideals represent those of the circuit, and the athlete only when his life is built around his sport. Some of these subcultures and the stereotypes they create are often circumstantial stages rather than permanent and definitive ones. You will also meet men who can simultaneously engage in and represent two or more groups at the same time.

THE ORIGIN OF GAY GYM CULTURE

It all began with the ancient Greeks and the most powerful male ideal ever conceived: the Greek ideal (Chapter 2), a body type characterized by well-defined muscles that are developed without being overly bulky, symmetry in the upper and lower body, and an absence of body fat. The ancient Greek statues of Apollo and Hermes reflect the ideal, and the writings of Homer, Pindar, Plato, and Aristotle expound on it. As if that was not enough, the ideal was furthermore represented in the surviving paintings and drawings of ancient Greece. But intellectual debate about and artistic representation of the ideal did not stop in ancient Greece; without looking too hard we can find the ideal in the writings, sculptures, paintings, and now movies, videos, and photographs of modern times.

Ancient Greek gym culture is of special interest to us because homosexuality was as much a part of it then as it is today. Likewise, when we speak of the Greek ideal, the propagation of the ideal and homosexuality are inseparable and historically well documented, albeit barely explored. The Greek ideal is truly more complex than its physical representation; for the ancient Greeks it was the embodiment of mind and body in perfect harmony. Very similar ideas today are shaping a growing mind/body-conscious gay subculture.

The Greek ideal reemerged in the paintings and statues of the Renaissance: this set the stage not just for gay gyms to sprout up in the 1970s, but for modern male body culture as we know it to take its shape. In Victorian times, the sport of bodybuilding revived, and this led to the gym becoming a modern social institution.

Historical and anthropological discussions of gay gym culture are important for two reasons. First of all, it helps us understand how history created the stereotypes that are defining us (for better or for worse) today. Second, when I looked into the evolution of these ideals, I have found that homosexuality was not at all divorced from the creation of these ideals; rather, it was a founding factor. As I will discuss in the next three chapters, gay gym culture is a modern phenomenon with ancient and homosexual roots. Homosexuality has not just influenced gym culture—it is heavily responsible for its creation.

THE BODY BEAUTIFUL

When we look at the influence of homosexual males in terms of body and gym culture, we realize that gay gym culture influences gay/queer history as much as it does mainstream history. A mistaken generalization about gay gym culture is that it is the result of the media's overindulgence on the body beautiful, and that gay men have become the puppets of Madison Avenue. This is not entirely false, but it is neither entirely true. I have pondered the media's involvement from a less critical and more historical and anthropological perspective and will discuss the influence of "muscle media" (Chapter 4) as it has shaped modern culture. In pondering the influence of media on gay body culture, we must recognize that gay men are a big part of Madison Avenue. Sure, the media is a driving force, but it is often driven by gay men. We are not the victims or the puppets of Madison Avenue—we as a cultural force are quite often the puppeteers.

The most obvious product of gay gym culture is the developed male body—the body beautiful. Most commentaries about the gym and gym culture, whether in admiration or critique, ask the question: Why are gay men obsessed with the body? Where did this preoccupation with the body beautiful come from?

There is no simple and definitive answer; the answers are many. The body, and the way it is perceived, changes dramatically from person to person, from one age group to another, and from one subgroup to the next. The only wrong answer to the question, which unfortunately is also the most common one, is the one that assumes a single answer for everyone. As we will learn, the body and the gym have very different meanings for a twenty-five-year-old circuit boy (Chapter 9), than they do for a forty-seven-year-old muscle bear (Chapter 10), or a seventy-nine-year-old retired professor (Chapter 11).

Yet the body is central to every group regardless of how different its members are from one another. The body, specifically the homoerotic body, is also central to homosexuality; this is another parallel we find throughout history. This is an important parallel because it is at the core of gay identity. For this reason the male body is the nucleus of this book, and I place quite a bit of emphasis on the larger picture that the male body represents. Not your body, or my body, but how the male body has been viewed and perceived at different times in history and how these representations connect to both modern body culture and the gay agenda. In doing so we will discuss the body as it has been represented in marble, photographs, and paintings (among other media), and, more importantly, what place these representations take in our minds to form ideals and subcultures built around those ideals (Chapters 2, 3, and 4).

The history of the body beautiful in relationship to homosexuality has important lessons for queer people. We know that men have been pondering its influence for the last 2,500 years. We also know that the appreciation of the male body beautiful by other males has traditionally been linked to homosexuality. In this history we can chronicle much of the struggles for acceptance that homosexuality has encountered. Today, the body beautiful represents for the most part a superficial celebration of beauty, but in the recent and ancient past, the same images represented symbolic and political statements. In this book I examine the role that the body beautiful and its representation have had in gay history and gay liberation (Chapters 2, 3, 4, 5), as well as the impact it continues to have in modern gay society (Chapters 5-12).

CRITICS

On the desirability scale in gay culture, the muscular male has little competition. He rules. He has become the ultimate object of desire. The gym-built man has the kind of power that sometimes even money cannot buy or education bestow. Wielding that kind of power guarantees examination, and this is one of the reasons gay gym culture has generated the criticism it has. Another factor is that gym-built men have become a large and very visible group. The criticism, often based on myths created by those for whom gay gym culture is foreign or threatening, is problematic for two reasons: much of it is based on erroneous information and anecdotal evidence, and it continues to mystify gym culture rather than understand it.

One cannot argue with the points some writers make about the superficial nature of gym culture. But these writers assume that the gym is about nothing but aesthetics. Is the gym about aesthetics? Absolutely. In Chapters 6, 9, and 10, I will entertain you with just how much, but the gym is also about a lot more. I will discuss the role that aesthetics plays in modern gay life and examine both our superficial motives and our deeper ones. Any psychologist will tell you that our most superficial motives are always tied to our deepest ones. This is where it gets interesting, as understanding those superficial aspects will help us understand the more complex ones. In this book you will meet young men for whom the gym represents only an outlet to bigger biceps, but you will also meet others for whom the gym and athletics have been the catharsis for life-changing and sometimes life-saving experiences.

Because the only precedents to such a subculture in which homosexuality and the gymnasium were interlinked were documented in ancient Greece, and because today thanks to gay social critics the only literature on the subject is more negative than positive, it is imperative that we examine gay gym culture objectively. The philosophers and writers of the ancient world celebrated the body and the importance of a mind-body connection, while also discussing the downside of too heavy a preoccupation with the physical. Their modern counterparts fail to see what's beyond the physical and focus only on what's wrong with gym culture rather than what's right with it. In this book I aspire to take a balanced approach between the two points of view.

Conclusion

In urban gay America, the gym is now an extension of gay social (and sometimes professional, recreational, and political) life. It has, as in ancient Greece, become the nucleus of gay life. If in the 1970s and 1980s the gay gym became a social institution for gay men in gay ghettos, now it has become a social movement without walls or borders. The gym is fast becoming the *third space* for a lot of gay men of all age groups. The gym has largely replaced for many gay men the bars and happy hours so popular among gay men in the 1970s and 1980s.

By taking into account the sociology, psychology, anthropology, and history of gym and body culture, in this book I examine the gym and its subcultures beyond the realms of exercise and fitness and explore it as the social institution it has become. I aim to have a frank discussion about ideals and stereotypes that shape modern thought. This book is intended to be an intelligent and unbiased dialogue that discusses both the benefits and drawbacks of the subculture and concurrently examines some of the biggest myths of muscle boys entertained by those who are not familiar with the men of the gay gym.

Chapter 2

Greek Gym Culture and the Greek Ideal

In gay culture today, athletics and the pursuit of a sculpted physique are increasingly becoming an important aspect of our social and cultural lives—so much so that a backlash has arisen against gym and body culture. Many modern gay writers and social critics have spent quite a bit of ink condemning what one suggests has contributed to the "fall of gay culture."[1] Michelangelo Signorile in *Life Outside,* Edisol Wayne Dotson in *Behold the Man, The Hype and Selling of Male Beauty in Media and Culture,* and Daniel Harris in *The Rise and Fall of Gay Culture* have dedicated much of these titles to bashing gym culture and the cultivation of the body.

As someone who had spent over a decade working closely with gay gym culture, I found the previous books and similar articles inaccurate and misleading for two simple reasons. One, their collective deductions are heavily based on anecdotal evidence coupled with recently acquired folk wisdom, and almost completely ignore 2,500 years of history and philosophy. And two, if we examine how social structures are built and the societies in which they thrive, it does not take a rocket scientist to figure out that a social trend like gay gym culture is a direct, albeit complex, result of the rise and liberation of gay culture—not its downfall.

To better understand and explain human phenomena—gay gym culture, in this case—we must examine its foundation as well as the social structures that created it. That is exactly what this chapter and the next one are about. The foundation and social structures of gym culture, athletics, and the male body ideal prevalent today are found in one place: ancient Greek gym culture. When we look to Greek art and literature we find that twenty-first-century gym culture is nothing

Muscle Boys: Gay Gym Culture
Published by The Haworth Press, Taylor & Francis Group, 2008.
doi:10.1300/6034_02

new: Greek society of 2,500 years ago shared many similarities to today's gay gym culture. There is enough evidence in the art and literature of classical Greece to substantiate that not only was the Greek gymnasium a male-centered institution, but a homosexual male-centered one. During the Golden Age of Greece (around the fifth century BC), the high point of Greek culture and influence, the Greek gymnasium became prominent. The culture of the Greek gymnasium, where Greek athletics were born, the Olympic games were set in motion, and the male body ideal was conceptualized, can be best described as one that was largely made up by men who were sexually and romantically interested in and involved with other men.

Now that gay gym culture has become a substantial cultural and social group in modern society, it is constructive to examine the differences and parallels in Western culture of two very similar male-centered *physique movements* that thrived 2,500 years apart. In this chapter I discuss Greek homosexuality, take a look at how Greek homosexuality, often intertwined with gym culture, was documented by the literature and art of classic Greece, and explore the homosexual-influenced social structures that were founding aspects of the Greek athletic ideal and the Greek gymnasium.

GREEK HOMOSEXUALITY

Documented Western gay history can be said to have begun with the Greeks, and many of our ideologies and belief systems about sex, homosexuality, and the body can be traced to the same origins. Countless references in art and literature have taught us that homosexuality in ancient Greece was as much an accepted and normal behavior as heterosexuality. The Greeks did not even have nouns that described the sexual orientation of men; it was simply normal for men to love or lust after young men as much as after young women. Sexuality did not include the divisive, distinctive definitions that it entails today, and homosexuality most definitely did not have to be explained or excused. In explaining on a superficial level why homosexuality during the fourth century BC was such an accepted culture, K.J. Dover said it best: "They accepted it because it was acceptable to their fathers and uncles and grandfathers."[2] It's a simple, yet legitimate explanation, which could very well be used in understanding the prevalence of exclusive heterosexuality today.

In fact, because of the higher status that men had over women, male-male relationships were in many cases considered not only noble but also superior to male-female relationships. Heterosexual relationships served the purposes of procreation and the family, but the union of two males often represented higher love. In *Symposium,* one of Plato's most renowned books, the philosophers discuss Eros between men:

> Those sectioned from a male pursue the masculine; because they are slices of the male, they like men while still boys, delighting to lie with men and be embraced by them. These are the most noble boys and youths because they are by nature the most manly. Some say they're most shameless, but they're wrong: they don't do it out of shamelessness but out of boldness and courage and masculinity, cleaving to what is like themselves. A great proof: actually, it is only men of this sort who, when they grow up, enter on political affairs. When they reach manhood they love boys, and by nature pay no heed to marriage and the (be)getting of children except as compelled to it by custom and law; it suffices for them to live out their lives unmarried, with one another. So this sort becomes wholly a lover of boys or a boy who loves having lovers, ever cleaving to what is akin. When the lover of boys . . . meets his own particular half, they are then marvelously struck by friendship and kinship and Eros, and scarcely willing to be separated from each other even for a little time.[3]

Pederasty

Greek homosexuality has, for the most part, been studied as the by-product of the pederast type of relationships that according to historians were common in ancient Greece. The pederast relationship was typically made up of an older man or *erastes* (lover) who would undertake a male youth as his lover or *eromenos* (beloved); aside from consuming a sexual and romantic relationship would also become his mentor and ensure his education. A common mistake many people make when discussing pederasty in Greek homosexuality is to assume that these relationships were, unlike today, only of a sexual and brief nature, and again, unlike today, not a way of life but a rite of passage. However, enough evidence suggests that quite often, homosexual relationships involved two men of or about the same age, and, as I will discuss, akin to relationships today, including everything from brief sexual encounters to lifetime partnerships. Furthermore, even if we do accept the pederast theory as dominant, it should be noted that Greek males evolved through different stages of the pederast relationship, from "beloved," *eromenos* during youth to "lover," *erastes* during mid- to late stages of adulthood, which means that they were practicing homosexuality throughout their life and not briefly or as a rite of passage.

An important fact that until recently many classic and queer-studies historians often overlooked is the strong connection between Greek homosexuality and pederasty to Greek athletics and the ancient Greek gymnasium. The most notable exemption has been made recently by Thomas F. Scanlon, author of *Eros and Greek Athletics,* in which he discusses authoritatively and in depth the fusion of homosexuality and Greek athletics.[4] Pederasty involved education, and as I will explain, gymnasia were a significant component of education. Homosexuality/pederasty and ancient gym culture were for the Greeks part of the same equation; one cultivated the other and vice-versa. As Cicero himself pointed out, albeit perplexed, "to me at any rate this custom [of pederasty] seems to have been born in the gymnasia of the Greeks . . . where those loves are unrestricted and permitted."[5]

Literature

We can further our understanding of homosexuality, the beauty and appeal of the male athlete, and the ancient Greeks' body ideal by referring to some of the most respected and oldest literature of Western civilization, that of Homer, Pindar, and Plato. The magnitude of athletics and of the male athlete can be found in the oldest surviving literature in Western culture, the *Iliad* of Homer. Aristotle gave Homer his highest praise as a poet, and Alexander the Great is said to have always had at hand his copy of the *Iliad.* Yet, as David Sansone writes in *Greek Athletics and the Genesis of Sport,* the larger-than-life blind poet did not find it unsuitable to dedicate the twenty-third volume of the *Iliad* to the athletic contests held at the funeral of Patroclus.[6] (The twenty-third volume of the *Iliad* also relates in part the legendary love affair between Achilles and Patroclus, as the games were held to honor the love and passion that Achilles felt toward Patroclus.[7])

The poetry of Pindar (518-438 BC), considered by the most serious scholars to be the greatest Greek lyric poet who ever lived, was so revered that when Alexander the Great destroyed Thebes in 335 BC he ordered his warriors to spare only the temples and Pindar's house. Pindar's surviving work, the four books of the *Victory Odes,* were composed to celebrate the champions of the athletic games. Although Pindar's interest in the games was mostly philosophical, he nevertheless dedicated much of his life to writing about the physical prowess of athletes, and in so doing gave us a peek into the significant roles that athletics and male athletes played in Greek culture.

From the Greek gymnasiums emerged the young wrestler Aristocles, who had made a name by twice winning the wrestling prize at the Isthmian Games. He would eventually become better known by his ring name, a name that would come to describe one of the most influential thinkers of all time: Plato. Most scholars have agreed that Plato was exclusively homosexual, and some maintain that aside from the Bible, Plato's *The Republic* has influenced Western thinking more than any book.[8] In the Socratic dialogues of *The Republic,* Plato and his counterparts discuss the steps necessary in finding the ideal harmony of the soul and of the state. In their ideal republic, the philosophers discuss the importance of gymnasiums in the education of heroes. The following is a dialogue between Socrates, Glaucon, and Adeimantus as narrated by Plato in *The Republic*:

> And what shall be their education? Can we find a better than the traditional sort?—and this has two divisions, gymnastic for the body, and music for the soul.
>
> True.
>
> Shall we begin education with music, and go on to gymnastic afterwards?
>
> By all means.
>
> And when you speak of music, do you include literature or not?
>
> I do.[9]

In *Symposium,* Plato enlightens us on the fusion of pederasty and gymnasia, as well as the antagonism, that like today, gay gym culture receives from less enlightened people:

> In Ionia and many other places where people live under the rule of the barbarians [pederasty] is considered base. This is shameful to the barbarians because of their tyrannical governments, as are also philosophy and the passion for athletics (philogymnasia). For, I suppose, it is not in the interest of the rulers that the subjects have high thoughts, nor strong bonds of friendship or society, which Eros most especially above all these other practices is accustomed to create.[10]

Male homosexuality was so prevalent in the culture of classical Greece that romantic relationships between men abound in the mythology. The most famous is certainly that of Zeus and Ganymede: the legend holds that Zeus, ruler of Gods and men, fell in love with Ganymede, a beautiful Trojan prince and son of King Tros. Zeus, after giving Tros a gift, abducted Ganymede and carried him off to Olympus to be his cupbearer and concubine. The abduction is represented in numerous vase paintings of the classical period. In literature, Homer recites the myth in the *Iliad.*[11] And in Olympian 1, an ode dedicated to Hieron of Syracuse (victor of the horse race, 476 BC), Pindar describes the love affair:

> It was then Poseidon seized you,
> overwhelmed in his mind with desire, and swept you
> on Golden mares to Zeus' glorious palace on
> *Olympos, where, at another time, Ganymede came also*
> for the same passion in Zeus.[12]

There are also many documented cases of same-sex relationships and love affairs in the scriptures of Greek history, many of them including Olympic athletes and other men involved in the culture of the Greek gymnasium. According to John Boswell, the Zeus-Ganymede type of abduction became a ceremonial model of male-male relationships in ancient Greece that established a legal relationship between male lovers. In his words, this practice had:

> . . . all the elements of European marriage tradition: witnesses, gifts, religious sacrifice, a public banquet, a chalice, a ritual change of clothing for one partner, a change of status for both, even a honeymoon.[13]

Probably the boldest account of homosexuality in classical Greece involving male equals was that of the Sacred Band of Thebes, a feared militia of 300 warriors composed of 150 pairs of male lovers. Created by Gorgidas, a Theban military leader, in 378 BC, the Sacred Band had crucial impact in many battles and was not beaten until the Battle of Chaeronea in 338 BC; in describing what made the band so powerful, Plutarch reasoned:

> For tribesmen and clansmen make little account of tribesmen and clansmen in times of danger; whereas a band that is held together by the friendship between lovers is indissoluble and not to be broken, since the lovers are ashamed to play the coward before their beloved, and the beloved before their lovers, and both stand firm in danger to protect each other.[14]

Art

The art of antiquity is priceless in our evaluations of Greek culture because before the invention of photography, magazines, and later television and movies, the various media of art acted as the main channel, outside of language, of exchanging cultural standards and ideology. These media were for the most part limited to literature, sculptures, and paintings.

In Greek art, the intense fascination with muscular male athletes and the male body suggests not only the homoerotic impulses of the artists but the demand created for such art by the men who could afford it. Hypotheses abound about the possible meanings of artistic representation at different times in history; therefore we can only speculate how art was perceived 1,000 or 2,500 years ago. However, by the standards of Western modern-day culture, and even those of premodern Europe, it would be not only naïve, but virtually impossible, to try to divorce the Greek male nude from some sort of erotic symbolism, and—more to the point—one of homoerotic manifestation.

One might argue that art was not homoerotic, that it was simply *homocentric,* or male-centered (as have many classic scholars). But it is obvious that the graceful youth takes on erotic representation because the subject is not representative of power alone but of male beauty. It is in this beauty that we can also see the fusion of masculine and feminine features that has always been a defining aspect of gay culture. And while the homocentric theory might make a good argument for the sculptures, when it comes to the vase paintings depicting graphic sexual acts between the athletes and other men, it cannot be further argued that homosexuality did not play a vital role in Greek athletics and other cultural life (see Figure 2.1). Figure 2.1 illustrates two Greek males having anal sex, and this photo in particular has been printed and discussed in many books discussing Greek homosexuality as simply a homoerotic image. What many, if not most, scholars have failed to identify is that given what we know about

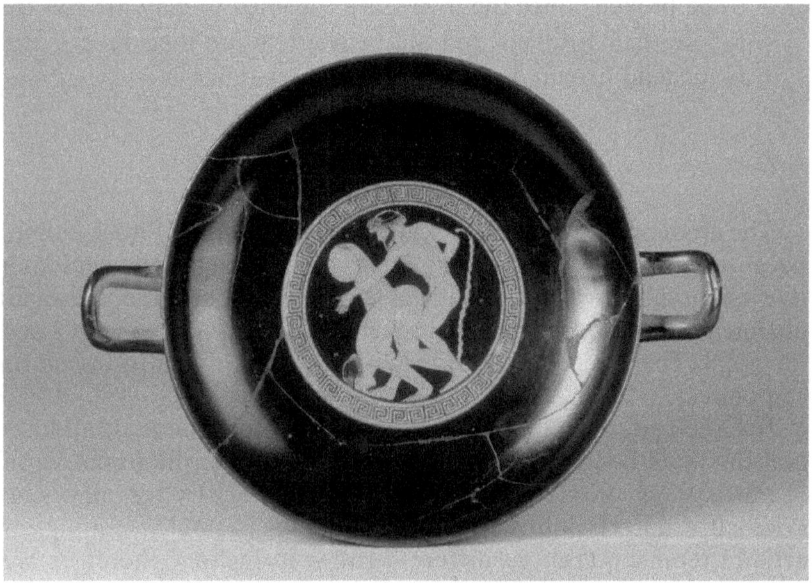

FIGURE 2.1. Red-figure kylix decorated with a homoerotic scene by Briseis Painter (5th Century BC), Ashmolean Museum, University of Oxford, UK/The Bridgeman Art Library.

Greek athletics the image is without a doubt sexual intercourse between an athlete and his trainer. The muscular definition of both males indicates that both were athletes and the cane and toga in the background are possessions of the bearded male, and indicative that he was a trainer. In the Greek gymnasiums, as Figure 2.2 illustrates, only the trainers, who were typically older, wore beards and togas and walked around with a cane that was sometimes used to discipline the young athletes (see Figure 2.2).

The sculptures and vase paintings, in short, document what was the object of desire to the Greeks. In both we can see the naked beauty of the young men. Young but postpubescent men, fully grown, developed muscles, yet with hairless bodies and pretty faces depicting youth and beauty. What's more, outside of literature it is in the vase paintings that we can uncover the obvious prevalence of homosexuality.

A more interesting question might be to ask how the art under discussion could not have been homoerotic. After all, women were not citizens or considered the equals of men in ancient Greece, and were not allowed in the gymnasium or at most competitions. To even suggest that the same art was created for or aimed at a female audience would be unreasonable. The art of ancient Greece representing the male nude was created solely for the enjoyment and scholarship of men.

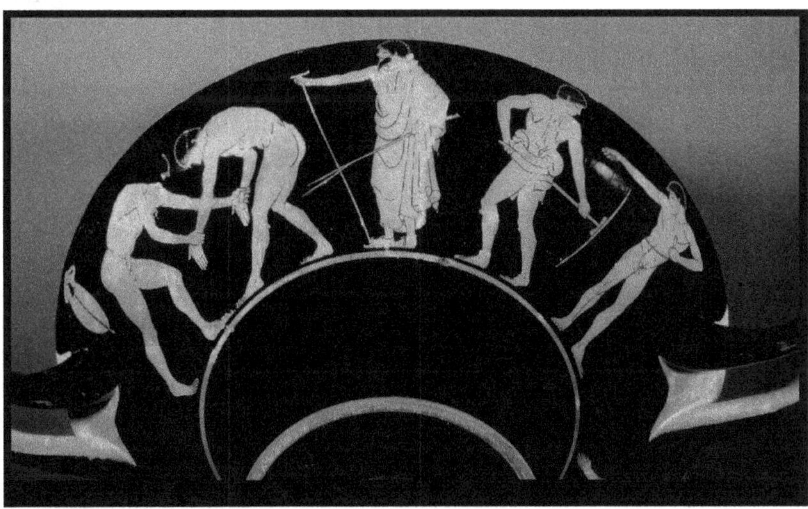

FIGURE 2.2. Attic red-figure kylix depicting athletes training (5th Century BC), Ashmolean Museum, University of Oxford, UK/The Bridgeman Art Library.

THE GREEK IDEAL

In the sculptures of sixth-century BC, the *strongman,* characterized by being overly built, stocky, and sometimes fat, often a boxer or wrestler, prevails. In the fifth-century BC we see a shift toward the *graceful athlete,* who is leaner, defined, typically young, and almost always pretty (see Figure 2.2). In gay culture today the ancient strongman could be compared to a modern-day muscle bear; the graceful athlete would appear more like a lean, but not overbuilt circuit boy or the leaner type of athlete such as a swimmer, runner, or cyclist. It is this more athletic, yet sculpted, and muscular but lean body that would set the Greek body ideal that prevails today, of which Michelangelo's *David* gives us the perfect example (see Figure 3.1). The statues and red-figured vase paintings started projecting muscularity and leanness; the shift was from strength to physical beauty and grace.[15] It is this shift that documents the birth of the beautiful male celebrated in art and subsequently of the Greek ideal. At the same time, a more sexual undertone was presented, emphasizing homoeroticism in ancient Greek art. E. Norman Gardiner, a historian writing in the nineteenth century who noted the differences of the subjects in the red-figure vase paintings, makes clear that "If strength is the key note of the sixth century, that of the fifth is the union of strength and beauty."[16]

No other ideal has been more influential in shaping men's bodies than the Greek ideal. The reasons gay gym culture has exploded are many, and we will discuss these in detail later, but at the core of these reasons is the pursuit of an idealized, sculpted body. The male body ideals of today, with a few exceptions, are for the most part identical to the Greek body ideal—a body that most readers would recognize as developed, muscular, lean, and absent of fat and imperfections.

The body ideal warrants discussion, not for its merits or for its flaws, of which it has plenty, but for the enormous influence it has had and continues to have on gay culture and ultimately gay history. Rather than take a stance for or against the body ideal, my goal is to examine the beliefs, systems, and assumptions surrounding an idealized body, further discussing its history and influence in today's gay gym culture as well as male pop culture. Whether we like it or not, perfect specimens of the body ideal have come to symbolize gay men. Gym culture—today or twenty-five centuries ago—revolves around precisely the same body ideal. In a change from previous stereotypes, in the past few years the muscular and built male is more and more becoming synonymous with the gay male.

Although this book focuses on gay male culture, it is also important to make a distinction between the conceptualized ideal bodies of men and those of women. The female body ideal was created through the objectification of women–by men–and has fairly enough been protested by many cultural critics, feminists, and writers. Although nowadays women objectify the male body in the same way that men have objectified the female body for millennia, they have been doing this on a significant scale only since the onset of the women's movement: the past thirty years account for only about 1 percent of the period under discussion. The critical difference is that women did not create the male body ideal, because it was already there: it was created, cultivated, pursued, and celebrated by men for 2,500 years before women would have a say in the matter. More to the point, because homosexuality was a widespread practice by the culture of the Greek gymnasium as the Greek body ideal evolved, and because men who had sex with men were the ones who conceptualized and refined the ideal, by and large the Greek ideal can be defined as a homosexual concept.

To understand the origins and foundations of the body ideal it is imperative to look at Greek religion and education. The body ideal has its roots in the ancient religions; to the Greeks beauty and skill were considered gifts from Zeus, so to posses such virtues represented a connection with the gods. Simply put, the more beautiful, the more godlike. Often the games and festivals of Olympia were in honor of Zeus as well as other Greek gods. The Greek gods Eros, Hermes, and Heracles (and sometimes Apollo) were, according to Greek literature, the main patrons of sport, and their statues were common at the stadiums and gymnasiums.

An athlete's victories or defeats were attributed to the blessing or curses of the gods. It was because of Greeks' religious beliefs and fears that honor and morals played such an important part in sports. In fact, much of the ethics of sports still in practice today evolved from the religious aspects of ancient athletics. The games were offered to the gods, and, as Gardiner explains, to be unfair or dishonest would be a sacrilege to the gods.[17]

In *The Perfectible Body,* an exemplar book on the developed male body through history, Kenneth R. Dutton studies contemporary examples of the developed male body and traces them to their cultural antecedents, noting that:

> As Greek religion evolved, the gods came to be envisaged less as divine beings in anthropomorphic form than as idealized representations of perfected humanity. . . . And its most potent exemplar was, for the Greek artistic mind, the muscular male athlete. . . . The athlete modeled himself on the hero of myth, and in so doing took on much of the symbolism of heroic stature.[18]

Aretē

Intelligence and academics today are viewed in Western culture as mutually exclusive from physical beauty and athleticism. The cultivation of the body is regarded, at best, as play time and more often as narcissism. In Western civilization, and especially academia and previously aristocracy, the separation between brains and brawn has been so severe that to use the two in the same sentence has, for the most part, regrettably been reduced to an oxymoron. As David Sansone writes in *Greek Athletics and the Genesis of Sport:*

> We find it much harder to accept the fact that sport plays so great a rôle in Greek literature. The reason is that we tend to regard sport and literature as belonging to very different levels of experience: one is part of our serious cultural life, the other is merely a form of entertainment or recreations. But for the ancient Greeks, clearly no such distinction existed.[19]

The Greeks, as Sansone points out, found no such divisions necessary: to them, aesthetics and athletics were considered part of a good education. Although they had a physical body ideal, that ideal was not exclusively physical but part of a holistic pursuit of perfection, of excellence, or what they called *aretē*.

Aretē represented in the Greek mind the maximum marriage of mind and body, a concept in which they fervently believed. *Aretē* to the Greeks was the embodiment of personal excellence, of an idealized *perfected* state of being that included academic and athletic achievement as well as character and physical beauty. Because of *aretē,* young Greek males strove for knowledge, athletic skill, humility, honor, and a certain body ideal. It is in *aretē* that we find the strongest similarities to the mind-body fitness today. Later I will discuss in detail the many reasons gay men today are involved in the gym, but an overwhelming number of us are seeking a stronger and healthier mind-body connection.

To thoroughly understand *aretē,* the evolution of athletics, and the Greek body ideal, we must also recognize that the main schools of education in ancient Greece were literature, music, and physical education—and that all three were considered of equal importance. The Greeks placed such an emphasis on developing the body along with the mind that two of the first gymnasiums, the *Academy* and the *Lyceum,* were named for two schools of philosophy—those of Plato and Aristotle.

Aretē reinforced the Greeks' drive to excel in competitions, in everything from athletics and literature to music, drama, and beauty. The relaxed poses of the Greek statues of fifth-century BC project the humility and dignity that were a goal of *aretē* education: the body firm and upright, but relaxed, the head gazing down—a man modest, athletic, lean, and muscular but not overbuilt. In short, the statues show men who are beautiful yet lacking arrogance. The vase paintings document training, competition, and performance, so in this we can observe the skill and prowess of the athletes. In the vases we can see more aggression, but this is of course during training or competition, in which such aggression is desired. What's more, the vase paintings indicate the celebration and high status of the boy victor and male athletes in general in the same way that modern media celebrate male athletes and supermodels (see Figure 2.3).

Ever since gay liberation, we find a similar competitive element in modern gay men, ranging from the boardroom to the weight room. At the disapproval of social critics who disregard gym culture as nothing more than the pursuit of narcissism, gay men have, as a group, become quite competitive in athletics and bodybuilding while staying at the vanguard of mind-body fostering.

The humility and modesty factors of *aretē* teach us that we still have much to learn in modern gym culture. Humility and modesty are not defining characteristics of many muscle boys today; we need to remember that the cultivation of the body goes hand in hand with the

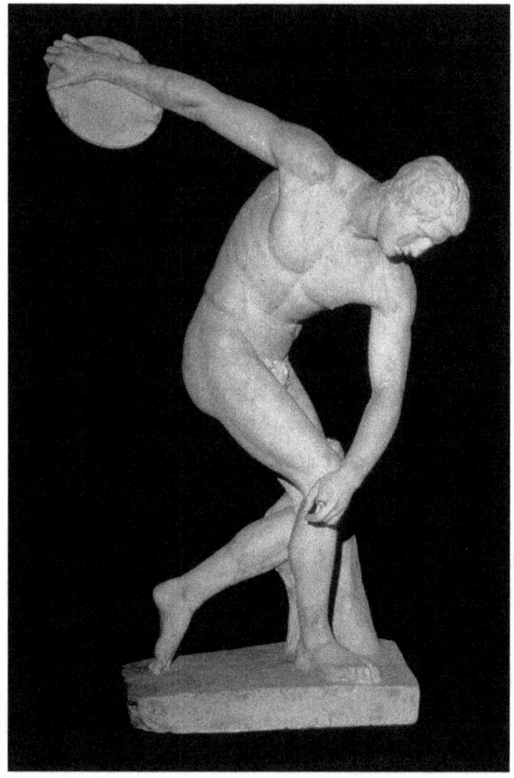

FIGURE 2.3. Discobolus (marble) by Myron (fl.c.450 BC) (after), Location Unknown/Ancient Art and Architecture Collection Ltd./The Bridgeman Art Library.

cultivation of the self. I strongly believe that for this to occur, we need kinder social critics and a community that's not only more involved but also more supportive. From the advances in mind-body medicine we are learning that the Greeks were quite right about the mind and the body not being two separate entities. And, as the cultivation of the body *alongside* the mind becomes supported by modern science and a more acceptable social phenomenon, concepts such as *aretē* arise, and we can better pursue wholeness. The fact that such virtues were encouraged as part of education indicates that to the Greeks—as is true with many of us today—these virtues were not intrinsic; they were something to aim for. Like any ideal, it should be noted that *aretē* was not the standard; the concept, like the sculpture, was an aspiration, not the reality of most young Greek males.

The Greeks left us with countless references of the body ideal, the male nude, and homosexuality, all of which seem intertwined—very much like today. In Greek culture we can observe and study these dynamics in the surviving sculptures, vase paintings, and literature of the classical period. The art—beautiful, remarkable, and at the same time simple, the literature just as beautiful and a bit more complex—all sum up the history as we know it, and clearly represent a strong—homosexually influenced—gymnasium and body culture.

THE GREEK GYMNASIUM

The Olympic games originally were not just about sport and competition, but were large festivals for the citizens of the *polis,* very similar to today's Olympic games, Gay Games, or other events involving athletic competitions, such as the World Series or the Super Bowl. A large portion of the citizens were involved in athletics and competitions. As Gardiner points out, before athletics became professional in the fourth century BC, Greece was a nation of athletes.[20] The Olympics, which started as a foot race, grew to the level it did because of the large participation of the citizens of Olympia and other Greek city-states.

As athletics and competition evolved in Greece in the fifth century BC, two things happened. First, games started becoming more of a spectator sport; second, training took on a more important role and moved from the stadium to the gymnasium. The stadium was the place of competition and battle, whereas the *gymnasium* and the *palaestra* (wrestling school) became the training grounds for the men of the *polis*. By contrast, the reverse of what happened in the fifth century BC is taking place in modern culture. Over the past few decades, more and more people are getting involved in competitions and athletic events on a recreational and nonprofessional level. Correspondingly, more and more people are going to the gym, whether to enhance their sport or to look and feel better.

The art and literature of ancient Greece substantiates just how much male athletes were cherished, and, without a doubt, the victors of the gymnasium were the most prized boys. The elevated status of the gymnasium boys came in part because of their physical beauty and skill, but also because they were often to become warriors—they were considered heroes in training. Because athletes and warriors both enjoyed heroic status, their social circles and lives frequently intertwined—socially, sexually, and romantically.

At the gymnasium, men of all ages would train in the sports of throwing the discus, javelin, running, wrestling, jumping, pentathlon, and weight lifting. Because of their belief that a healthy, strong body was linked to a healthy mind, the gymnasium, very much like today, played a crucial role in the upbringing and socialization of males. The Greek gymnasium was more than a training center. Scholars such as Dover, Gardiner, and Sansone, among many others, agree that it was the social meeting ground for well-to-do male citizens of the *polis*. In this, we again find resemblance to modern gay gym culture, as the gym has become a nucleus of the social lives of urban gay men today. Aside from being the Greeks' artist studio, it was common for men to visit the gymnasium simply to socialize or to watch the athletes train. It may seem peculiar to us, but it becomes clearer as we examine the dynamics of the Greek gymnasium.

One of the most fascinating yet perplexing facts of the Greek gymnasium and of athletic competitions was the custom for men to exercise and compete completely naked. The word *gymnos* in Greek means "naked," and the word *gymnasium* translates to "a place where men exercise naked." One of the first rooms at the entrance of the ancient gymnasiums was the *apodyterion,* or undressing room. While nudity is not allowed in modern gyms, one thing is clear: the heavier the populace of gay men, the more skin we see. At the gay gyms of today, men are not exactly naked, but many come tremendously close. In the gay gyms that surfaced in the gay ghettos in the 1970s it was common for men to work out in nothing but shorts and shoes. As I point out in Chapter 5, there is at least one reference to a gay gym in San Francisco during the same decade where members were allowed and many actually worked out naked. Similarly, if we look at other institutions and events where gay men congregate outside of the gym, such as gay pride events, circuit parties, nightclubs, and bars, we also find more skin than we would at heterosexual hangouts.

The nudity in Greek training and athletics has perplexed a great many scholars, for there seems to be no rational explanation for it. However, when we view the gymnasium as a homosexual hangout, it becomes a bit clearer. As Dover explains:

> The gymnasium as a whole or the wresting-school . . . provided opportunities for looking at naked boys, bringing oneself discreetly to a boy's notice in the hope of eventually speaking to him.[21]

Although there are a couple of references suggesting that the reason for the nudity was aerodynamics, they are vague, and the concept would have been to the Greeks mere speculation rather than science. Aerodynamics in sports focus on minimizing air resistance or drag by wearing skintight outfits or very little clothes so that the athlete can move faster through space. However, because the type of foot races that were common in the fifth century BC do not really provide enough air resistance to cause a significant amount of drag—as it would in cycling, for example—and because humans can run just so fast, such aerodynamic principles truly benefit only the most modern elite athletes.

Even if the Greeks found enough evidence that a nude body would move faster through space, that might justify the nudity in competitions, but it would not explain the nudity during training at the gymnasium or the dress for the chariot races. Other scholars have hypothesized that the nudity's purpose was to instill discipline in the male trainees, which makes a bit more sense given the sexual attitudes of the time. Along with the many vase paintings depicting athletes training or in competitions, we find many that explicitly depict the male athletes engaging sexually with one another as well as with their trainers and other men (see Figure 2.1). As most men would agree, too much of a preoccupation with sex can keep us from other pursuits, and if the vases are at all representative of the sexual mind-set of the time, then the need for self-control and discipline when it came to athletics is more than evident. Even today, although research has shown that sex the evening before an athletic event will not affect performance, many athletes and coaches still believe in waiting until after competition.

The notion of self-discipline and chastity in Greek athletics is reinforced by another attention-grabbing practice by at least some of the men of the Greek gymnasium: temporary *infibulation*. In females infibulation refers to removing the clitoris and sometimes even sewing shut the labia. In males it is less permanent and refers to tying a string around the foreskin on the penis.

The young Greek men of the gymnasium would (only at times) infibulate themselves for training and competitions. As much as we know about infibulation, it is mainly a form of chastity, supposedly to prevent an erection in the infibulated male. Another possible explanation of the temporary infibulation is that it makes the penis look smaller. A large penis was not as desirable to the Greeks as it is to many men today, so perhaps they used the strings to make their penises appear smaller and more attractive, very much in the way that some men today use cockrings to make their bulges appear larger. There is not enough representation in the vase painting to suggest that infibulation was all that common, so we don't really know just how general the practice was. Regardless, temporary infibulation is another possible example of just how widespread homosexuality was in Greek athletics, because women were not allowed at the gymnasium or at most competitions, and only other males surrounded the male athletes. In any case, it was out of attraction or desire for other males that they were either avoiding erections or making themselves more attractive. Like some of the other practices and customs of the Greek gymnasium, we might never find out the extent and true objective of infibulation, but we do know that like other Greek ideals, *sôphrosyne* (the Greek virtue of self-control) was something to work toward, not something that already existed.

Besides the *apodyterion,* or undressing room, other rooms at the gymnasium included the *ephebion* (club room), the *elaiothesion* (oil store), the *konisterion* (dusting or powder room), and the baths.[22] The elaborate bathing rituals of the Greeks before and after exercise have inspired much debate among scholars. The biggest problem that scholars such as Gardiner have faced when writing about such bathing rituals probably stem out of the homophobic, longstanding beliefs in Western culture that such grooming practices were suitable only for women. In Gardiner's defense, we have to realize that he was writing in early twentieth-century England, a time when homosexuality was very much taboo, and a time that had not yet seen the full effects of the physique movement that was just beginning to take place. Again, by the standards of today, in which men in general have become accustomed to showering and grooming at the gym, such amenities would not seem out of place. In fact, the better health clubs and gyms of today have brought back the club room, introduced shops, and built lavish locker rooms with hot tubs, steam rooms, and saunas.

Although the Greek literature confirms that the gymnasium became known as the place for men to meet male lovers, in his otherwise levelheaded book Gardiner was bewildered on the possible use for some of the "extra rooms" at the gymnasium.[23] While we can only speculate whether sex took place at the Greek gymnasium, if we take a quick tour at the locker room of gyms today (both gay and straight), the probability does not seem so unlikely.

Attitudes toward the body and nudity in ancient Greece were similar to what they are in contemporary American culture. Even at the time of the Greeks, nudity was controversial to foreigners: the Romans, for example, found it degrading for men to exercise or compete in the nude. The Greeks, on the other hand, believed that to be ashamed to be seen naked was the mark of a barbarian. These differing viewpoints reflect modern-day attitudes, although not so extreme. Note the different attitudes about clothing and nudity in the United States versus those in Europe.

The confusion concerning nudity at the Greek gymnasium has arisen, at least in part, because until recently most scholars who have researched Greek athletics have completely separated Greek athletics from homosexuality. When we link the two as inseparable aspects of Greek social life, the nudity can be identified as a potential characteristic of homosexual behavior. As Scanlon points out: "Athletic nudity is one of the factors that undoubtedly fostered and was fostered by pederasty in Greece generally."[24]

Although I do not envision fully explaining nudity in Greek athletics, I have two possible, yet opposing, theories of its purpose. On one hand, it makes sense that since the mind and body were intertwined for the ancient Greeks, the nudity was then connected to a vision of wholeness or in the Greek concept of *aretē*. On the other hand, as I've mentioned before, the games were large festivals providing entertainment for aristocratic men. In the latter case, then, it could simply be that in part the nude athletes provided visual erotic enjoyment for the male spectators. This notion is not so farfetched when we compare it to gay urban nightlife; today gay men are entertained by go-go boys and male strippers at nightclubs or circuit parties and poured cocktails by buff, shirtless, sexy bartenders at gay bars.

I have a feeling that there is some truth in both examples. While it is true that the Greeks' body ideal was based on the noble aspects of *aretē,* education and sports were largely linked to their religion. We also know that they considered the male body to be an object of beauty and desire, and one can safely speculate that they objectified it as much, or more than we do.

In summary, the ancient Greek gymnasium was a nucleus of Greek homosexuality and homoeroticism. So much was this the case, that when referencing instances in which heterosexuality is the focus of eroticism involving male athletes, Scanlon refers to its occurrence as "a phenomenon that must have occurred ordinarily outside the precincts of gymnasia."[25]

Full Circle

> Cicero said that Greece had undertaken a great and bold plan, namely to have set up statues of Cupid and deities of Love in the gymnasia.[26]

When we compare modern gay gym culture with the culture of the ancient Greek gymnasium the similarities are so many that it seems as if we have almost gone full circle. We cannot possibly divorce homosexuality from ancient Greek athletics. To do so, and this has been done quite a bit, is to distort Western history. Taking into account the dynamics of Greek sexuality and especially homosexuality, we can see that the ancient gymnasium was at the heart of everyday homosexual social life. Of course, life then was very different from what it is today, but by modern standards the Greek gymnasium was for the most part what we would call a gay environment, remarkably akin to the modern gay gym.

Sure, some things have changed; Nike, the Greek goddess of victory, is now an athletic garment label and a fashion statement. Some things have not changed at all, the high-protein muscle-building diet introduced 2,500 years ago by Dromeus of Stymphalus, an Olympic victor and trainer, is now more popular than ever. Twenty-five centuries ago, the male nude was commonplace; today, the male nude or seminude is everywhere in media and increasingly at social events such as nightclubs and circuit parties. During the Greek Golden Age it was the men of the Academy and other Greek gymnasiums who would model for the sculptures of Apollo and Hermes and reveal for centuries to come what the body of a Greek god looked like. Today, out of gymnasiums everywhere emerge the male supermodels, actors, and porn stars that represent and determine male body-image standards—both gay and straight—for modern men. Emerging from any of the popular gay gyms in West Hollywood, San Francisco, New York, and Miami—displaying the familiar characteristics of the Greek gods—are collectively considered the hottest men in gay culture. In addition, akin to ancient Greek gym culture, an almost *athletic nudity* is becoming commonplace in modern festivals and "social competitions" such as gay pride events, circuit parties, and athletic events.

Because of the dynamics of classical Greek sexuality, the culture of the influential Greek gymnasiums is more analogous to contemporary gay gym culture than to the conventional, straight-male-dominated gym. The Greek gymnasiums were known not just as a place for men to build their bodies or train for sports, but also as a social center and a place where men could go to find male lovers. Platos' Academy was such a social and sexually charged—homosexually to be specific—place, that men enthusiastically admitted to being there just to socialize or gaze at the boys. As I will discuss in the remainder of this book, the exact social and mating possibilities are one of the most influential forces shaping gay gym culture today. Many gay men today would agree with an ancient Greek poem by Theognis of Megara which boldly states: "Happy is the lover who after spending time in the gymnasium goes home to sleep all day long with a beautiful young man."[27] Twenty-five hundred years later, Erôs is once again in rendezvous with athletics and homosexuality in a place called *gay gym culture.*

Chapter 3

The Fall and Rise of the Gym-Built Body

In this chapter I discuss both the artistic representation of the male nude and the gym-built body, showing how they go hand-in-hand, and the strong connection they have to homosexuality. The "full circle" I mention in this chapter began in the representation of the male nude, which receded during the Dark Ages, and made a comeback during the Renaissance. Such "fall and rise" of the gym-built body and the prevalence of gym culture occurred over three notable periods spanning approximately 2,000 years.

First, the fall of the Greek empire did away with the gymnasiums where men built, appreciated, or displayed their bodies. Gymnasiums became obsolete starting with the rise of the Roman Empire and would not again become conventional until almost 2,000 years later in the late nineteenth century. Because of its homoeroticism, the male nude was for the most part censored after the fall of the Greek empire. The Catholic Church, once it came into power in the fourth century, also kept him clothed, outlawing the pagan festivals and practices significant to Greek athletics and sports. Second, the Italian Renaissance gave birth to artistic and philosophical representation of ancient Greek culture and ideals, including the athletic ideal. During the Renaissance the male nude was rediscovered and once again celebrated in art form. And third, and of most consequence, in the late nineteenth century, a return to the Greek ideals of cultivating the body was introduced with a new sport: bodybuilding.

THE FALL: THE ROMANS AND CHRISTIANITY

The celebration of the male body as well as the prevalence of homosexuality started changing with the fall of the Greek empire and

Muscle Boys: Gay Gym Culture
Published by The Haworth Press, Taylor & Francis Group, 2008.
doi:10.1300/6034_03

the rise of the Roman Empire, soon before the emergence of Christianity. Although homosexuality was prevalent in Rome, it was a subject of controversy. With the loss of Greek independence to the Romans in 146 BC, the Greek gymnasiums and the palaestrae that were not a part of Roman culture started losing ground. One of the main reasons for this is that the gymnasiums and palaestrae did not provide the grounds for training in the type of gladiator sports that were popular in Rome. A second reason is that the Romans viewed the gymnasiums and palaestrae of Greece with some contempt because of the nudity and its reputation for being a place where men could find men for sex. In fact, according to Plutarch, the enslavement of Greeks was blamed on the gymnasium and the palaestrae, because of the prevalent homosexual environment.[1]

The antigym-culture sentiment in Rome changed temporarily in AD 60 when Emperor Nero (AD 54-68) established Greek-style competitions in Rome.[2] Roman citizens met Nero's decision with some resistance, but then Nero's homosexuality was already somewhat controversial in Rome. Like many homosexually inclined men before and after him, Nero was interested not only in Greek athletics but also in the dynamics of the Greek gym culture, and of course in the male athletes of the gymnasium. While he was emperor, he held a public ceremony and married *Sporos,* a male Olympic athlete. Their wedding was celebrated in Greece as well as Rome.[3]

Although the sexual attitudes in Rome were definitely narrower than in Greece, there are many accounts which prove that sex and romantic relationships between men were not at all uncommon. In fact, there are many references of same-sex unions and love affairs involving the emperors and most respected citizens of Rome, such as Hadrian (emperor of Rome from AD 117 to 138) and Antinous, and Diocletian and Maximillian. Another example is that of Elagabalus (emperor of Rome from AD 218 to 222) and Hierocles, an athlete who is described by Elagabalus's biographer as his "husband."[4]

The documented cases of unrestricted homosexuality appear mostly during the early part of the Roman Empire; this started changing with the rise of the Roman Catholic Church. According to historian John Boswell, it was not until AD 342 that a "law forbidding same sex weddings" was instituted in Rome. This of course has its grounds in the emergence of Christianity during the fourth century; as Boswell points out, "At the opening of the century Christianity was illegal; by its close paganism was punishable by death."[5]

During the same century, in AD 394, the Roman emperor Theodosius, under force by the Roman Catholic Church, put an abrupt end to the Olympic games and all other pagan rituals. At the time of their death, the ancient Olympic games had lasted more than 1,200 years, longer than any known ceremonial event in Western history. The ban on the Olympics lasted for more than 1,500 years, until they were revived in the late nineteenth century.

At this time, the fully clothed sculpture was introduced and the nude became for the most part obsolete. When it was used, the nude started to take a different form and to represent shame and evil. It would increasingly be used in art only to represent those in the dwellings of hell. Kenneth R. Dutton makes a brilliant observation:

> Apart from the Damned, only three portrayals of the unclad human body exercise the imagination of the medieval mind: Adam and Eve, the crucified Christ, and St. Sebastian.[6]

For almost 2,000 years after the fall of the Greek empire, the human body in Western civilization was covered and concealed. The naked body was associated with sin and evil; it was seen as a dammed vessel, something dangerous that could lead us into temptation. So strong was this belief, that punishing the body through self-flagellation was a popular practice among Roman Catholics during the Dark Ages and early medieval times. The naked body represented, to the medieval mind, something to be ashamed of. It was not to be celebrated.

THE RENAISSANCE: THE HOMOEROTIC BODY REDISCOVERED

Beginning in the fourteenth century and lasting into the seventeenth century, a humanistic revival of classical influence saw the birth of modern science and a blossoming of the arts and literature that had been in hibernation since the classical period of Greece. It was during this time, the Renaissance, that the male body was rediscovered and once again portrayed and celebrated in sculptures, paintings, and literature by, among others, those who became known as the Italian masters: Michelangelo, DaVinci, and Caravaggio.

Through his magnificent paintings, his statue of David (see Figure 3.1), and other sculptures, Michelangelo carved the first layer off an old ideal, as much of his work was based on reconstructing the art of antiquity. The measurements of the limbs and body proportions of his famous *David* were taken from ancient Greek statues.

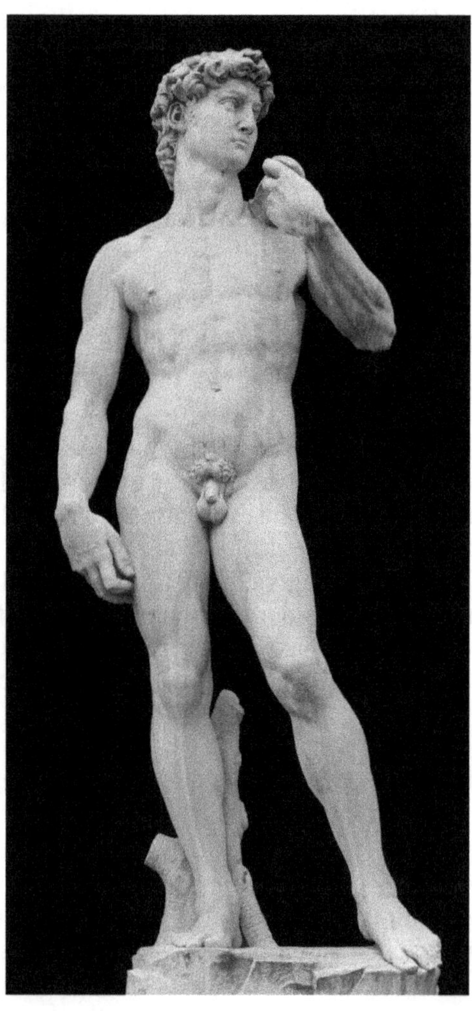

FIGURE 3.1. Statue of David, Michelangelo. © iStockPhoto.com.

One of history's most famous homosexuals, Michelangelo was not the only man in love with the male body. Leonardo DaVinci, too, had the same fascination. When he was not painting, sculpting, or inventing, he was busy painting and sketching the anatomy of the male body. Historians believe that Leonardo was also gay: when he was twenty-four he was arrested along with several male companions on charges of sodomy. He never married or had relationships with women, and it is assumed that Salai, his protégé, a younger man who appears in his sketches and who lived with him for more than twenty years until his death, was his longtime lover. He is regarded as one of the first anatomists, and his work greatly influenced modern medicine. One of his most famous drawings, *Vitruvius Man,* depicts the naked perfection in the human body. For centuries to come, his many anatomy studies were also of great value to other artists who would use them to better represent their work.

Without some sort of divine representation, works of art involving the male nude would not have been allowed by church and state. Furthermore, although the homoeroticism is obvious in many, the idea that a painting could represent erotic symbolism was not only forbidden but also dangerous to the artist.

Michelangelo's *David* became the measure by which a perfect man was measured, and the image of modern man began to change. However, the clothed, concealed, shameful body was, at this point, a 2,000-year-old convention, and difficult to break. It wasn't until the dawn of the twentieth century with the initial stages of modern bodybuilding that a true renaissance of the built male body began to occur.

BODYBUILDING: BUILDING THE MODERN IDEAL MAN

"Strongman" acts were popular entertainment venues in the eighteenth and nineteenth centuries, and often were part of a circus ensemble. Such acts typically consisted of feats of massive strength such as bending steel pipes, breaking chains, lifting colossal amounts of weight, even performing a somersault while holding a heavy barbell. Like other circus acts, it was a freak show. The typical strongman was built very much like the strongmen of classical Greece: big, burly, heavy, hairy, and husky, and by most modern standards, unattractive. What made them a spectacle was not physical attractiveness—it was their gigantic, brutelike appearance and massive strength (see Figure 3.2). Although men were interested in watching strongmen acts, it is also clear that most men who watched them were not at all interested in modeling themselves after the modern Brutus. On the other chromosomal end, while women were also part of the audience, for the most part, the strongmen did not represent an object of desire to them. That all changed at the end of the nineteenth century with Eugen Sandow.

Sandow, a vaudeville strongman, wowed his audiences not just with incredible strength (the purpose of the show), but also, according to his past and recent biographers and the many journalists who wrote about him during his career, with the "body of a Greek god," (see Figures 3.3, 3.4, 3,5, and 3.6).

LOUIS CYR,
POLICE GAZETTE CHAMPION HEAVY LIFTER
OF THE WORLD.
CHAMPAGNE'S STUDIO. No. 8 Hurd St., Lowell, Mass.

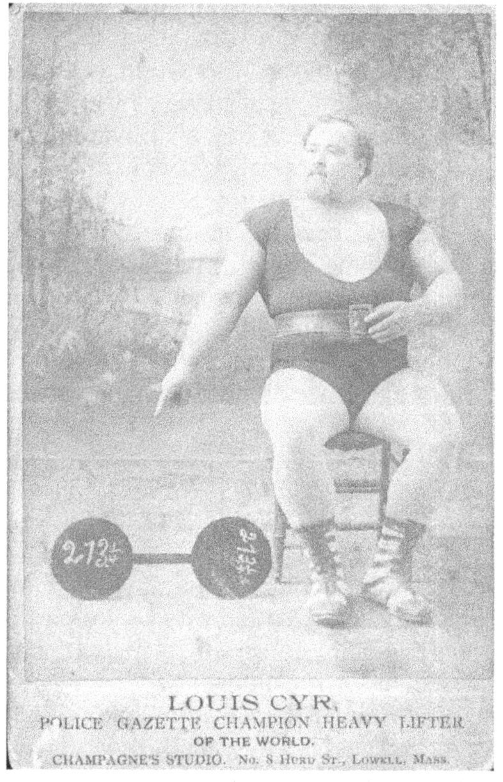

FIGURE 3.2. Louis Cyr, famous nineteenth-century strongman, Cabinet card (1900). Courtesy of The Magazine Archives, San Francisco.

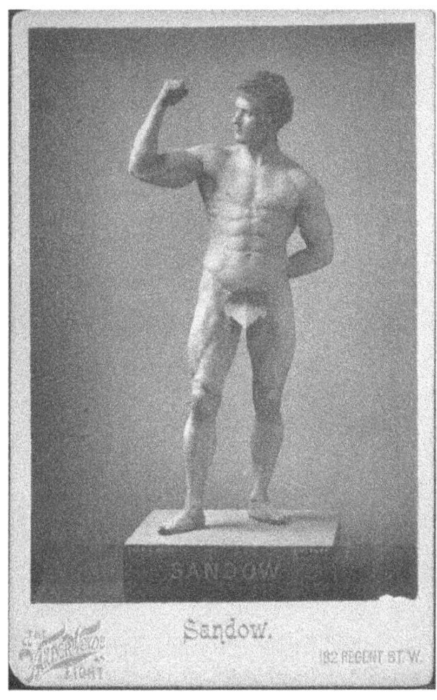

FIGURE 3.3. Eugen Sandow, father of bodybuilding, by Van der Weyde, Cabinet card (1894). Courtesy of The Magazine Archives, San Francisco.

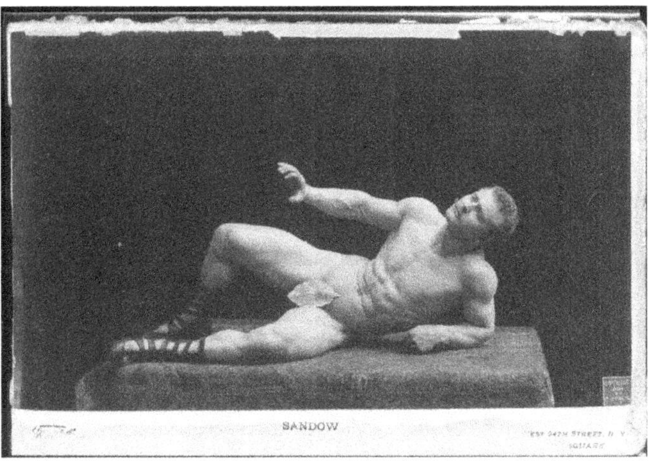

FIGURE 3.4. Eugen Sandow, by Falk, Cabinet card (1894). Courtesy of The Magazine Archives, San Francisco.

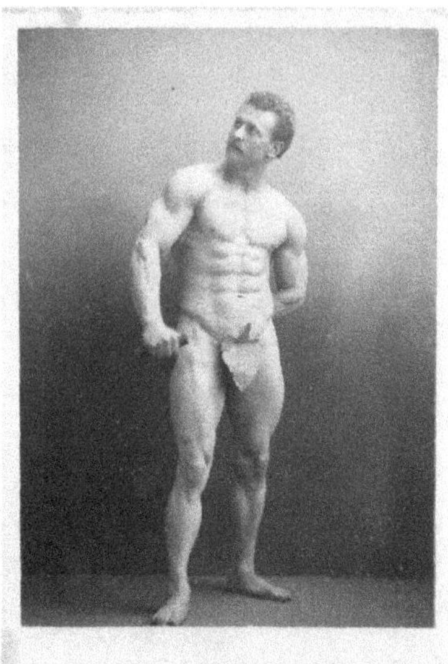

FIGURE 3.5. Eugen Sandow, by W. Brooks, Cabinet card (1915). Courtesy of The Magazine Archives, San Francisco.

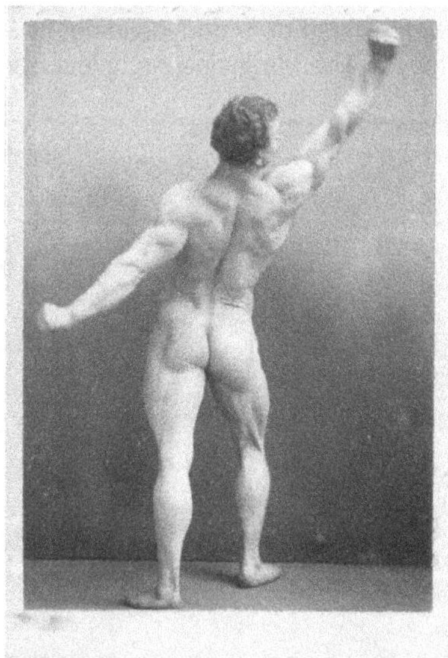

FIGURE 3.6. Eugen Sandow, by W. Brooks, Cabinet card (1915). Courtesy of The Magazine Archives, San Francisco.

Sandow received such a positive and sensational reaction to his sculpted body that he quickly realized he could capitalize not just on his strength but on the way he looked. His performances became less about strength and more about the display of his muscular physique. The sport of bodybuilding was born.

Technically speaking, Sandow was not the first bodybuilder. As an antidote to the sedentary lifestyles that were the norm to the upper classes, a small movement of physical culture had been started in 1812 by Friedrich Jahn in Germany, spreading later to Europe and eventually to America.[7] Although, by the mid-1800s there were gymnasiums in most large cities in Europe and America, it was a relatively small movement. Sandow merely popularized the sport and became its poster boy.

Eugen Sandow was born Friedrich Wilhelm Müller on April 2, 1867. In his late teens he adopted the stage name that would not only bring him wealth and fame but would revolutionize the image of modern man. With a background as an acrobat and gymnast, Sandow trained and built his impressive physique under the famed physical culture teacher "Professor Attila" (real name Louis Durlacher). Although Sandow did have incredible strength, it was, no doubt, his looks and chiseled body that wowed his audiences and ensured him prominence. Blond, blue-eyed, and handsome to the point of being almost pretty, he was sculpted like the Greek statues of antiquity. He was not built like the typical huge and bulky strongman of the nineteenth century. He was so muscular and defined that it set him apart from the average man. As David L. Chapman writes in one of the best and most researched biographies about Sandow: *Sandow the Magnificent, Eugen Sandow and the Beginnings of Bodybuilding:*

> Our fathers and grandfathers considered Sandow the epitome of masculine beauty–regally handsome and supremely strong. He seemed to be a Greek statue come to life, and they had never seen anything quite like him.[8]

Because of Sandow, for the first time in modern history the almost nude male body became not only somewhat acceptable but also, for Victorian dogma, the unimaginable: a positive image. This was no easy task given that the events under discussion were taking place at the height of the Victorian era. The nineteenth century had seen a strong rise of the middle class in Europe and America. Following the Civil War, people moved from the farms to the cities to pursue office jobs, start businesses, and enjoy the recreation venues and lifestyles that the cities offered. A thin body and pale complexion were the traits of the aristocrats and businessmen, who embodied the male ideal for the rising middle class. The very concept of cultivating the body for aesthetic reasons was completely out of context during the Victorian era—muscular bodies were associated with construction workers and unskilled labor, the anti-ideals of capitalism. Sociologically speaking, the early gyms were truly an anomaly of their times. It was with Sandow that muscles and beauty became once again part of the same equation. Although during his time he was clearly a sex symbol to both men and women, he was billed as "the strongest man on earth," a more appropriate and respectable title for Victorian times. For Sandow, breaking through Victorian prudery was like moving a mountain. The celebration, admiration, and more important, the acceptance of the uncovered male body could occur.

Today, the numbers of men built to proportions of Sandow are in every magazine ad, TV commercial, and billboard. In the 1890s he was such a sensation that, as Chapman tells us, princes and kings were routinely fans and part of his audience.[9] He was often described as a living Greek statue. Today, it is not uncommon for thousands of women and gay men to pack a Macy's department store for the appearance of an underwear model, or for gay men to line up fifty deep at a gay pride event to get an autograph from a Falcon porn star. We can only imagine how shocking and impressive to the average person Sandow was in the 1890s.

An avid businessman, Sandow built a fitness empire that would set precedence to the entire fitness world today. He built gyms (including the first that catered to working professionals and women), published several books and magazines, ran a mail-order business, sold and marketed home exercise equipment, and was instrumental in introducing physical education to academic curricula and military training. No level of personal success or wealth was greater than the impact that the industry he started would have on the average man. No other venue has altered the image of modern man more than the infusion of bodybuilding into popular culture. Bodybuilding eventually branched out into many different forms of a larger physique culture, which now amasses the whole array of fitness trends, many sports, and an ever-more-present male nude in media. This larger physique culture now includes every hard male body from the lean and tight underwear model to the oversized and steroid-enhanced Schwarzenegger type.

Most bodybuilding experts recognize Sandow as the "father of bodybuilding," and he is often credited in bodybuilding history books as such. However, a little known fact almost always gets omitted from any literary sources in which he is regarded: his bisexuality. According to Chapman, while Sandow was known to enjoy the company of women, "his tastes ran in other directions too."[10] When Sandow first came to America, presumably a male lover accompanied him:

> Crossing the Atlantic with him was Martinus Sieveking, described as Sandow's "great and inseparable friend." Sieveking was a Dutch pianist and composer who had known Sandow from his years in Belgium and Holland. The two men had been living together for some time, and when they arrived in New York, they again set up housekeeping on West Thirty-eight street.[11]

Sandow eventually married and fathered two children, although like countless married and presumably straight men then as well as today, his marriage did not do much to make him heterosexual—or monogamous.

Although the details of Sandow's infidelities and sexual escapades (of which there were apparently many) are trivial at best, we cannot ignore the fact that he was at least bisexual. From a gay historical standpoint, his homosexual interludes are much more interesting to us. This is true for two reasons: one, because we can show a pattern of bodybuilding and fitness as an accomplishment of gay culture; and, two, because in doing so we can pose the question: To what extent did Sandow's sexuality affect the shift from strength to male beauty that reshaped the image of modern man? Would Friedrich Wilhelm Müller have become Eugen Sandow if he were not erotically charged by the beauty of the male body? According to Chapman, Sandow claimed that the beautiful Greek statues of antiquity, which he admired as a child at the Italian museums, were his inspiration.[12] In Sandow, as in most gay and bisexual men, the connection between homosexuality and pursuing male beauty is more than palpable.

Psychologists and sociologists have been known to ponder the "cause and effect" relationship between homosexuality and bodybuilding. Is the bodybuilding lifestyle, associated with narcissism and its "obsession," if you like, with the male body a tangible trait of homosexuality? While this question can be as abstract as most queer theories, it nevertheless makes for a solid argument. The notion that the homocentric can lead to homoeroticism and to homosexuality is not unrealistic. Whether there is any merit to the concept remains contentious. However, if we are to answer this question with Eugen Sandow in mind, we can say that in the case of the man who founded the sport and accompanying lifestyle of bodybuilding, it most likely did.

As Sandow and bodybuilding became more popular, the wedding of muscles and masculinity would have a ripple effect, and very soon the words masculine and muscular would become synonymous, along with another word: heterosexual. What is paradoxical is that much of the concept of the ideal heterosexual man, then and now, was built around the school of Sandow, a man who was homosexually inclined.

If left to their own devices, tightly built social constructions will eventually deconstruct—except of course, when they are advocated by religious or political systems, in which case, logic and natural order seem to become irrelevant, as such systems continually fail to evolve with the times. It is no coincidence that the negative attitudes toward the male nude started to change during a period (around AD 1500) that has also been referred to as "the age of religious discord." The made-up *masculine-muscular-heterosexual-male* construction came up against a wall when both women and gay men started opening up their own gyms and weight training en masse during and following the gay and women's liberation movements of the 1970s. With the inclusion of women and homosexuality into the equation, the sturdy stereotype built around masculinity and perceived heterosexuality was not only challenged—it was broken. It is impossible to predict what kind of effect all of this will have, but one thing is for sure: not only is muscularity losing its association to masculinity and heterosexuality, but the tightly sealed definitions of heterosexuality and homosexuality are thinning every day.

It wasn't the strongman of classical Greece who became mythical and idealized—it was the less masculine, more graceful young male athletes of the hyperhomosexual Greek gymnasium. In modern times, it wasn't the hypermasculine and typically heterosexual strongman of the nineteenth century who would change the image of modern men—

it was the Greek godlike, homosexually inclined Sandow. In both cases, the homosexual and homoerotic fusion of masculine and feminine rises over the heterosexual and the hypermasculine.

Similar Shifts

The shift from strength to beauty that occurred from the sixth to fifth centuries BC took place once again, this time at the end of the nineteenth century. In antiquity, the shift from the strongman to the graceful athlete is a kind of mystery, although we do know that it took place at a time when homosexuality was prevalent in ancient Greece and more than likely the shift was influenced by its prevalence. Sandow is of interest to us for three reasons: One, because with him we can pinpoint exactly when and how the shift from strength to beauty occurred in modern times, as he was clearly the catalyst. Second, because from a gay historical standpoint, the shift was generated not by a heterosexual man as most people have assumed, but by one who was at least bisexual. Third, because as this shift occurred the developed male body became celebrated in a fashion that had not occurred since antiquity, encircling bodybuilding, fitness, and the whole gamut of the male body in media as a study of art and an object of beauty and desire.

Homosexuality and the representation and celebration of the male nude in its most eminent form—the gymnasium-built body—have historically been intertwined. As I have outlined in this chapter, from the Renaissance to the Victorian era, the rise of the male nude in artistic representation and the gym-built body in modern culture is a direct result of the influence and ideals of homosexual, bisexual, and homosexually inclined men: Michelangelo, DaVinci, and Sandow, to name just a few.

History indicates that the censoring of the male nude was often an attempt (a successful one at that) at censoring and criminalizing homoeroticism and homosexuality. Although these bold accounts of censorship and criminalization were the staple of the Dark Ages in Western culture, the reader should take note that similar occurrences of censorship and criminalization are not exclusive to Medieval times, and are currently the rule of the land in many conservative and especially religion-influenced (Judeo, Muslim, and Christian, to name a few) societies and sects today. The deeper layers and the role of the male nude as a political and social statement during the past 2,000 years is something that many modern cultural critics ignore altogether when they one-dimensionally write it off as superficial or narcissistic.

The nineteenth century saw an actual revival of athletics and the Olympics, as well as the onset of modern bodybuilding in which its founders were said to have the body of Greek gods. From the renaissance and the Victorian eras emerged a new modern male-body ideal, the gym-built body prevalent today, a direct heir to its Greek predecessor.

In the next chapter we will look at the gay men behind the controversial media campaigns that have standardized the male nude in contemporary culture. If we examine the works of art of ancient Greece and the Renaissance, we can find the similar characteristics that are overused today in Abercrombie and Fitch catalogs, Calvin Klein underwear ads, and other ads selling you everything from beer to vitamins. Today, the familiar characteristics of the Greek gods and Michelangelo's *David* that Sandow proudly displayed are everywhere: the bulging chests, the broad shoulders, the tight abdominal muscles, the rounded buttocks, the defined thighs and calves, the peaked biceps and full-fledged triceps, and, of course, the youthful-looking, hairless bodies.

Chapter 4

Muscle Media

The gym-built body that made Eugen Sandow famous also made him rare—few men of his time possessed the muscular symmetry of Michelangelo's David. A lot has changed: today the gym-built body is present everywhere and displayed not only by circus performers or strongmen as was the case 100 years ago, but by an ever-growing number of mainstream men from students and professors to waiters and accountants, and men in just about every profession, occupation, and trade you can think of. This phenomenon confirms the fact that a new ideal has risen: the muscle boy ideal. Although this ideal is not the exclusive domain of gay men, it is now more prevalent in gay culture than in any other subculture or cultural group. Ideals travel and incorporate themselves into the mainstream by several methods: of these, the most influential one is media—ranging from informative and medical to entertainment and erotica. In this chapter I take a look at how *muscle media* has propagated into the hands, eyes, and minds of modern men—while at the same time pointing out just how much the modern ideal of man has been influenced and shaped by gay culture. In doing so, this chapter traces the steps of homosexual influence in the various types of muscle media by which the muscle boy ideal has traveled in modern times: photography, print, film, television, and its most powerful vessel yet—the Internet.

The muscle boy ideal has become one of the strongest icons in gay culture—and it is rapidly becoming the standard for a substantial number of gay modern men. Interestingly enough, like many other trends that begin in the gay ghetto, it has also become the ideal for a great number of heterosexual men. We tend to believe that the rise of the gay muscled body is a result of gay culture assimilating into mainstream culture. To a very limited extent, this is true. However, if we look deeper into the evolution of physique culture in Western civiliza-

Muscle Boys: Gay Gym Culture
Published by The Haworth Press, Taylor & Francis Group, 2008.
doi:10.1300/6034_04

tion in the last century, we find that much of the rise of the muscular male body in mainstream culture is actually a result of gay influences in art, bodybuilding, and media. So what is really happening is another occurrence of what queer scholars refer to as the *gayification* of mainstream culture.

PHOTOGRAPHY: MARKETING THE IDEAL MAN

The invention of photography in the mid-1800s marked the birth of the most exciting new medium of communication since the printing press in 1450. As soon as the photograph was invented, photographic studies of the nude (mostly male) human body were produced (see Figure 4.1). By the end of the nineteenth century, bodybuilding was gaining popularity in Europe and America, and a small but growing trade of nude and seminude photographs of male bodybuilders sprouted up (see Figures 4.2 and 4.3).

One of the most impressive collections of Victorian strongmen and bodybuilder photographs is held by Robert Mainardi, author of the critically acclaimed photo book showcasing a fragment of his collection, *Strong Men: Vintage Photos of a Masculine Icon.* I spoke with Mainardi about the development and background regarding the trade of physique photography at the turn of the century.[1]

"It started out with [Eugen] Sandow and other people in that late 1800s period," Mainardi said, and also told me:

> They were basically stage strongmen and selling their photos in the lobby of the theater was just another way for them to make money. In the beginning it was sort of a theatrical development not so much a sport development. There was always an interest in physique development, but no one ever sought a way to commercialize it until the late 1890s when they found men who had personality and could go on stage. They would have lifting challenges, rivalries. This is mostly in England and the continent, until Ziegfeld brought Sandow to America, and created the sensation.

When I asked Mainardi about who created the demand for these photographs of seminude and nude bodybuilders he stated, "A lot of those pictures were meant to be sold to women, and were sold to

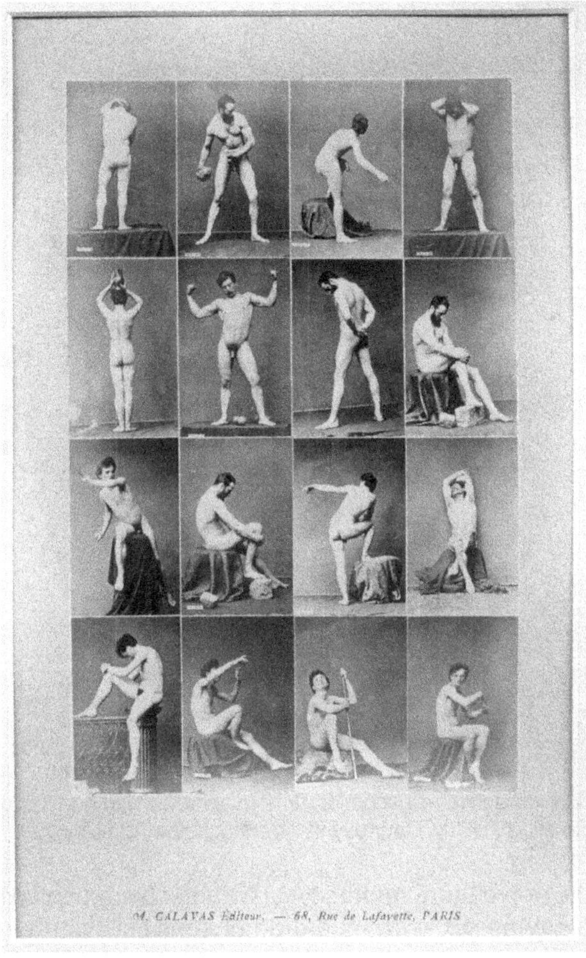

FIGURE 4.1. A. Calavas, French albumen print page of photographic figure studies from a folio (1865). Courtesy of The Magazine Archives, San Francisco.

women, although a lot of them ended up in the collections of men." When I questioned the sexuality of these men who fervently collected the first homoerotic photographs, Mainardi made an interesting point: "Until the development of the concept of homosexuality, a lot of gay men led straight lives." To gay and lesbian scholars, this fact is well known: before the word *homosexual* entered the mainstream vocabu-

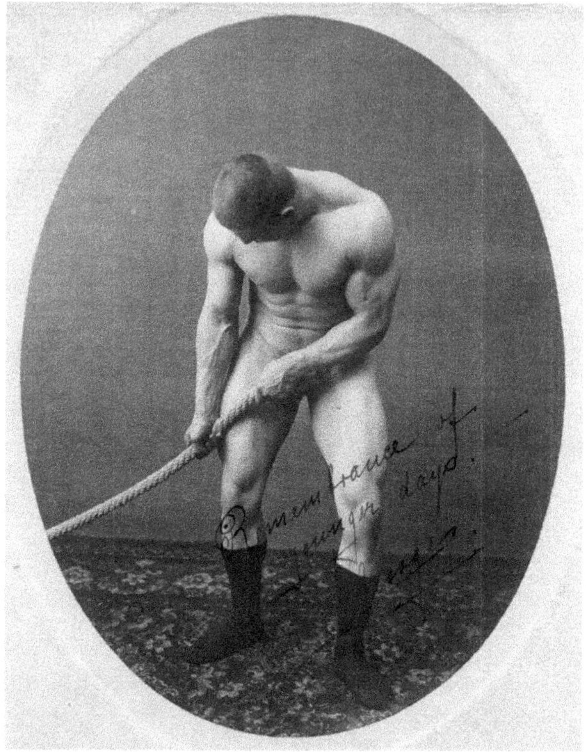

FIGURE 4.2. George Hackenschmidt, famous wrestler and bodybuilder; photographer unidentified (1900). Courtesy of The Magazine Archives, San Francisco.

lary and the pop culture mind-set early in the twentieth century, men who were having sex with men did not consider themselves gay or homosexual—something that still occurs today.

Yet, regardless of how collectors identified themselves sexually (or not), the trade of strongmen photography began clearing the way not just for homoerotic media but more importantly for homoerotic expression, as Mainardi agreed:[2]

> I think actually doing feats of strength, and breaking chains and bending nails, that went on for a long time into the 1920s and leading to the development of physique contests and also the [silent] movies . . . all had a big influence at the idea that you could look at a handsome men just because he was handsome.

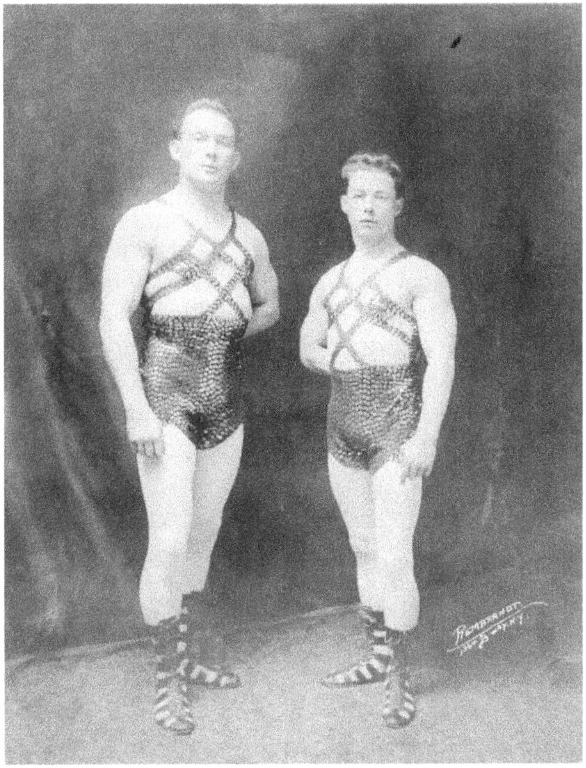

FIGURE 4.3. Roland Brothers, probably a vaudeville act, by Rembrandt Studio, NYC (1910). Courtesy of The Magazine Archives, San Francisco.

A visual history buff, Mainardi is also quick to point out that the representation of the male body as a human work of art is yet again turning another cycle:

> It does happen in cycles. Cycles when male nudity is absolutely forbidden and female nudity is the only acceptable artistic fashion; periodically it reverses itself. Now we're in the modern period where both are becoming acceptable, which is probably healthy. I think it was inevitable with the development of modern culture that this would happen. Because women had been commoditized for so long, it was just matter of time before people found out you could commoditize men, too. Throughout his-

> tory there have periods when the male physique was eroticized. Think of Renaissance Italy where they wore cod pieces to accentuate the genitals. That was accepted for a long time; that was the fashion.

Ultimately, the wedding of photography and physical culture made for the mass marketing of physical fitness and of what would become the modern ideal (see Figure 4.4). The new physique media became the main channel by which the modern male image would be redefined and become what it is today. Not only was the physique media redefining the modern male image, but as these different niches in media were making way, they played an enormous role in

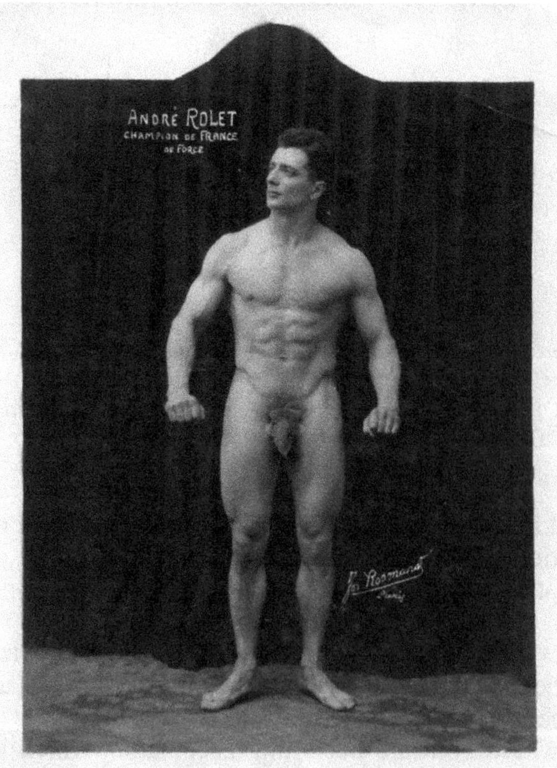

FIGURE 4.4. Andre Rolet, French bodybuilder (photo is marked "Jos Rosmand, Paris" on front but stamped "Photo Studio Armand Leflohic, Paris" on back) (1930). Courtesy of The Magazine Archives, San Francisco.

breaking down obscenity and censorship laws, which heavily influenced the rise and development of gay media as we know it. Eventually, the photography-bodybuilding duo would branch out into a colossal media kingdom of fitness, bodybuilding, photography, art, and pornography.

PHYSIQUE MAGAZINES

One of the most important milestones in the celebration of the male body was the introduction of the physique magazines at the end of the nineteenth century. Physique magazines were built around a new and very tiny subculture: *physical culture,* better known today as bodybuilding.

The first influential physique magazines were published in England and the United States. In July of 1898 Eugen Sandow published *Physical Culture* magazine in the United Kingdom, where he lived, which the always self-promoting Sandow would later rename to *Sandow's Magazine of Physical Culture.*[3] Although Sandow's magazine was quite successful during his lifetime, it was one of Sandow's American fans, fitness buff Bernarr MacFadden, who would have sky-scraping success with the publication of a series of bodybuilding and fitness magazines in America. The first and most notable was named (exactly like its European sister publication) *Physical Culture* magazine—which of course was no coincidence.

According to biographer Robert Ernst, MacFadden attended the World's Columbian Exposition, which took place in Chicago in 1893. At the Expo he was quite impressed and inspired by the classical sculptures on display, but one man in particular would have a mighty effect on MacFadden: the lead entertainer and presenter, Eugen Sandow. Ernst relates how Sandow "Fascinated young MacFadden, who donned tights and began imitating Sandow's poses as Hercules, Atlas, Ajax, and Samson."[4] The Greek ideal had worked its charms once more. Soon thereafter, MacFadden would launch a career in physical culture, becoming the most influential man in America in the field of physical culture for several decades.

The first issue of *Physical Culture* was published by MacFadden in March of 1899 and sold for five cents a copy.[5] By 1903 circulation reached around 250,000 copies in the United States and the United Kingdom.[6] *Physical Culture* was a publishing success even by today's standards. While MacFadden inspired many imitations, the span and success of *Physical Culture* has been superceded in recent decades only by the modern-day media empire built by Joe Weider (Weider Publications publishes *Muscle & Fitness, Flex,* and *Men's Fitness,* among several other popular fitness magazines).

Filled with articles on nutrition, fitness, bodybuilding, sex, and mind-health information, the physique magazines were also loaded with pictures of nude and seminude young males. These publications were basically bodybuilding and fitness periodicals and their objective, basically, was to promote and teach physical culture. But the magazines featured photographs of near-nude men that often had nothing to do with the editorial content. The near-nude photographs in *Physical Culture* and other physique magazines that followed were obviously there for visual pleasure and inspiration, which is why they became known as physique magazines. The magazines made it possible for men to appreciate and admire the beauty in other men—in private and at almost any time they wanted. For the first time in modern history, the male nude photograph could be as accessible as the closest newsstand and the privacy of one's mailbox. The physique magazines could not print frontal nudity, but came pretty close (many of the models were covered only by the classic fig leaf). MacFadden was known to pose in the nude or almost nude quite often and did so well into his golden years (see Figure 4.5). From the beginning, *Physical Culture* was setting the precedent not just for bodybuilding and fitness media, but also for gay erotica and pornography. Although the success of *Physical Culture* resulted in several other imitations being published, MacFadden, by far, led the industry.

At a time when homosexuality was illegal and any mode of positive expression about it out of the question, it goes without saying that the new type of men's magazine would have a devoted homosexual audience. The physique magazines became an outlet of unofficial gay media. Whether the magazines catered to a homosexual or heterosexual audience is truly less relevant than the fact that the male body and male beauty could be appreciated openly in print for the first time.

Physical Culture was so successful that MacFadden took male beauty a step further. He staged the first male beauty contests in modern times: the World's Most Beautiful Man contest in which young males would compete for overall physical beauty. Eugen Sandow had staged similar contests, but they differed in that they revolved more

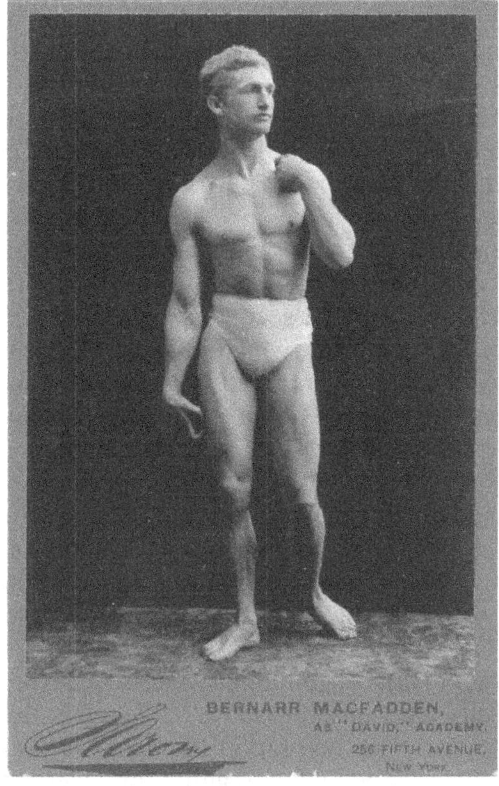

FIGURE 4.5. Bernarr MacFadden, publisher of *Physical Culture Magazine* and twentieth century fitness guru, Cabinet card (1900). Courtesy of The Magazine Archives, San Francisco.

around the physique and strength of the contestants and not about how beautiful they were. Eventually, MacFadden's contests evolved into the Mr. Universe, Mr. America, and Mr. Olympia bodybuilding competitions. The concept of men competing to be the best looking set the stage for the male beauty pageant that would become a popular part of gay culture. These include the overwhelmingly successful physique competitions at the Gay Games and the International Mr. Leather and International Mr. Bear contests—or other competitions you can attach the "Mr." prefix to. Make no mistake: these contests in every way are beauty pageants for men, whether they are judging the most beautiful bodybuilder, leatherman, or bear, the only thing that changes are the physical characteristics that make up the ideal in that specific subgroup.

Although many were happy about the introduction of physique magazines such as *Physical Culture,* others were not. Especially opposed were members of the Society for the Suppression of Vice which considered the magazine and its content immoral, simply because of its near nudity and a suspicion that it catered to homosexuals (which, intentionally or not, it did). In October of 1905, MacFadden was getting ready to open the second annual *Monster Physical Culture Exhibition* in New York, which featured physique contests for both men and women among other fitness-related races and activities. The event generated a large amount of publicity and controversy. The Society for the Suppression of Vice found the promotion posters lewd and obscene largely because they featured women in tights and men in loincloths, and MacFadden was arrested. The sensationalism of the arrest made for great press, and the case was widely covered by the media. Although MacFadden was found guilty, the court did not impose a penalty, and the show was a huge success largely because of the free publicity surrounding the arrest.[7]

The case was only the beginning of MacFadden's lifelong struggle against obscenity and censorship laws. Two years later, he was arrested again, over a story that ran in *Physical Culture*. This time he was not so lucky: after being found guilty for material the court considered "obscene, lewd, and lascivious," he was sentenced to two years in prison and fined $2,000 (a fortune in 1907). Outraged, MacFadden took the case all the way to the Supreme Court. When the Supreme Court refused MacFadden's appeal, he took it a step further. Through a campaign that he promoted in *Physical Culture,* MacFadden and his readers flooded the White House with petitions for a presidential pardon. MacFadden's brawny influence on the American public was successful: in 1909 President Howard Taft gave MacFadden a pardon.[8]

Challenging the law, albeit unsuccessfully and unknowingly, was MacFadden's greatest contribution to gay culture and media. He set precedents for gay pioneers in successfully challenging similar laws with the same type of magazines. More important, the cases would send a positive message to millions of Americans who were starting to believe for themselves that magazines like *Physi-*

cal Culture and the homoerotic images that it celebrated were acceptable.

Publicly, Bernarr MacFadden was heterosexual. Anecdotal evidence, however, suggests that his interests tended in other directions. In addition to several books and two romance novels, MacFadden was known to write articles for his magazines under "various pseudonyms of both sexes." Although he married unsuccessfully several times, he believed that marriage "was a human necessity . . . successful men nearly always married, . . . Its only purpose was procreation . . . and . . . denounced sex for pleasure." For an iconoclast in the full sense of the word, a man who was not very religious and so overly interested in worshiping the male body, his public philosophy that the sole purpose of marriage was procreation is curious. It could very well indicate that MacFadden simply did not enjoy sex with women; one of his wives referred to him as "a chaste Galahad" and in marriage he even "proposed separate bedrooms or at least separate beds." This is interesting, given the fact that he was busy creating, sponsoring, and promoting contests to find the "World's Most Beautiful Man."[9]

Charles Atlas

The winner of the World's Most Beautiful Man contest staged by MacFadden in 1921 was a young and handsome Italian by the name of Angelo Siciliano. Siciliano would also win America's Most Perfectly Developed Man contest the following year (also a MacFadden production) and would eventually become another icon of physical culture under his new stage name: Charles Atlas (named after the Titan from Greek mythology). Convinced that Atlas would win every time, MacFadden discontinued the contests. Atlas, however, was only starting to build an empire on his looks, body, and training methods.

Charles Atlas built a fitness empire largely through his mail-order business. From a queer historical perspective, his marketing methods were interesting. His advertisements boldly stated that you could go from being a "sissy" to a "real man." *Sissy* was the primary word in American vocabulary used to describe gay men at a time when the words masculine and homosexual were mutually exclusive. In his marketing campaigns Mr. Atlas seemed to describe the stereotypical "sissy" of his time—the homosexual. Was Charles Atlas attempting to make heterosexual men out of homosexuals? It's not a far-fetched idea when we realize that this occurred at a time when, not only was homosexuality considered an abnormality, but homosexually inclined men were actively searching for "cures" for their homosexuality. Although I don't doubt for a minute that one of Charles Atlas's direct target populations was homosexual men, one can only speculate on just how many gay men of yesteryear attempted his courses as a means to change their sexual orientation. This idea is not too outlandish, as even today when homosexuality is moving into the mainstream, many gay men seek to become more masculine through working out. Whether Atlas was directly marketing to gay or straight men, one thing is clear: his role in shaping the image of the ideal man into a muscle boy is profound.

Whether built by *Physical Culture* or Charles Atlas, muscular men, though not common, were becoming conventional by the 1930s and 1940s. The trend gained much momentum with the onset of World War II, as the military now routinely included fitness and weight lifting as an important aspect of training. At the same time, television brought moving pictures into American homes and the muscle boy ideal into American minds.

In 1948, a gorgeous bodybuilder named Steve Reeves won the Mr. America contest in Chicago (see Figures 4.6 and 4.7). From there he would win several other titles, including Mr. World (1948), Mr. USA (1948 and 1949), and Mr. Universe (1948 and 1950). He was so striking that soon Hollywood came knocking. Although Reeves starred in several hits of the 1950s and 1960s, he is more often remembered for his role in *Hercules* and *Giant of Marathon.* Steve Reeves was the first bodybuilder to become a movie star. With him the muscle boy had made it to the big screen and into the hearts of the American public. In more recent times, Arnold Schwarzenegger took over Reeves' role and place in Hollywood in the 1970s.

Beefcake and the Gay Media

After World War II, as muscle boys were becoming mainstream, so were their gay male fans. Although homosexuality was still illegal and punishable, gay men were beginning to organize. Two very important things happened in this period. One, as Charles Kaiser has discussed at length in his historical book, *The Gay Metropolis,* the presence of a

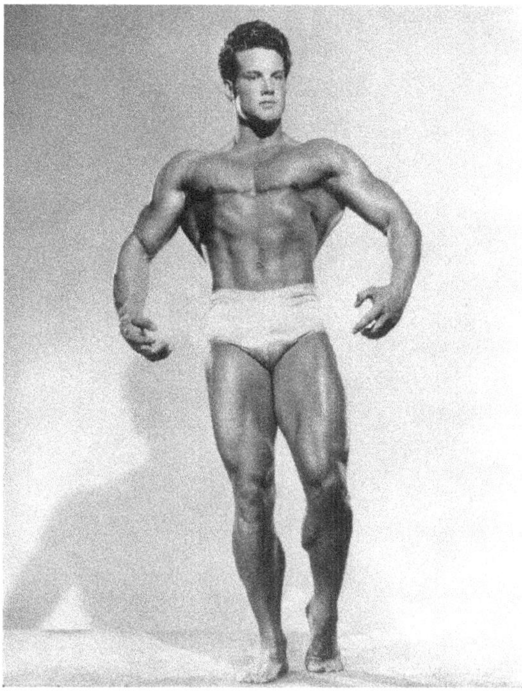

FIGURE 4.6. Steve Reeves, Mr. America 1947, and first bodybuilder to become a movie star, photographer unknown (1940s). Courtesy of The Magazine Archives, San Francisco.

huge number of gay soldiers started challenging the stereotype of the "sissy" homosexual, chipping away at the then-radical concept that men could be both masculine and homosexual at the same time.[10] Second, gay men started publishing their own physique and fitness magazines. The gay muscle boy was beginning to come out of the closet.

As bodybuilding became more popular, the number of young men available to display their physiques for the camera was greater than ever. More than willing to exploit the opportunity, gay photographers stepped up to the job. Studios were set up, mostly in cities such as Los Angeles and New York, and an underground trade of nude and almost-nude physique photography catered to an ever-increasing number of gay men. By mid-century, one gay man decided it was time for

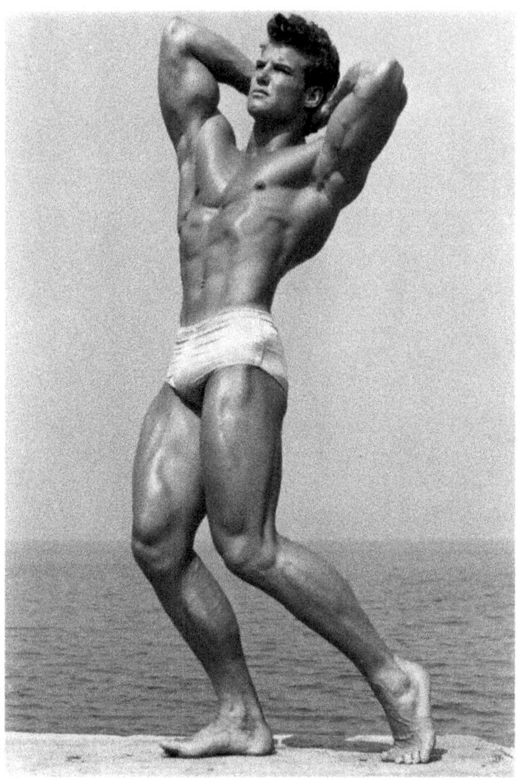

FIGURE 4.7. Steve Reeves, Mr. America 1947, taken on the Chicago waterfront by Tony Lanza of Montreal (1940s). Courtesy of The Magazine Archives, San Francisco.

gay men to have their own magazine. This man was Bob Mizer, and while there were many noteworthy gay photographers in this period such as Robert Maplethorpe and George Platt Lynes, none were as influential in the rise of a physique and gay gym culture as Mizer.

Bob Mizer started taking photographs of young men as a teenager in the 1930s and selling them in the back of men's lifestyle and bodybuilding magazines. His mail-order business did so well that he founded Athletic Model Guild (AMG), an attempt at a modeling agency for physique models. Although the agency was not a great success, the photography business was. By the late 1940s and early

1950s, the demand for Mizer's photographs had grown so much that when the U.S. Post Office started a campaign to "clean up" the men's magazines and his ads were pulled from them, he decided to start his own magazine: *Physique Pictorial*[11] (see Figure 4.8).

Dennis Bell, a San Francisco Bay Area photographer, acquired the estate of Bob Mizer after Mizer's death in 1992 and moved the AMG studios across the bay from San Francisco. Bell, a vintage physique aficionado, and the creator of posingstrap.com is an expert in the history of physique photography of the 1930s through the 1960s. In an exclusive interview for this book, Bell gave me a tour of the new AMG studios and we sat down to talk about Bob Mizer and the history of the studios. According to Bell, the original AMG studios started about 1945 in Mizer's mother's house. As his business grew, Mizer purchased the buildings on either side of her house, built a swimming pool, and used the three houses as a series of studios he called "the compound."[12]

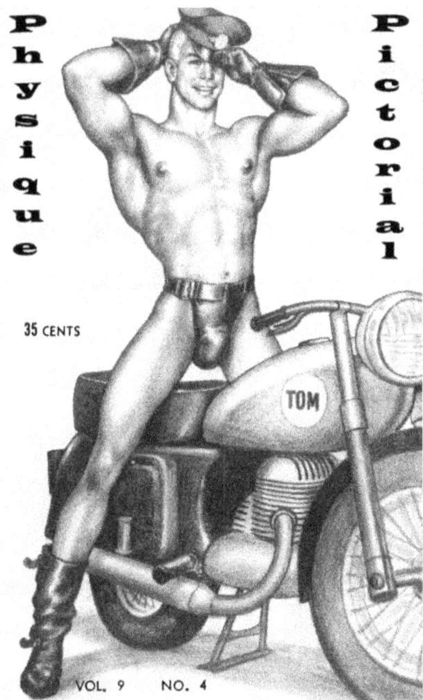

FIGURE 4.8. *Physique Pictorial* cover by Tom of Finland, Volume 9, No. 4 (1960). Courtesy of AthleticModelGuild.com.

Another interesting aspect about the photography of Mizer, supporting the thesis of this book, is the influence of the Greek ideal in his work. Many of his photographs and fantasy themes are representations of classic Greek art involving the male nude as well as homoerotic images from medieval and Renaissance periods (see Figures 4.9 and 4.10). Dennis Bell reported that Mizer became enchanted with Greek imagery when he went to Europe in 1951 and experienced firsthand the ancient Greek art on display at the museums. "He posed models to look like the statues," Bell said, adding that Mizer would use photographs he took in Europe of Greek temples and use them as background.[13]

> As things in Hollywood started getting into the sword-and-sandal movies, he drew on that quite a bit. Pictures of David, the thinker, and St. Sebastian tied up against the pole with arrows, are images that he did over and over.

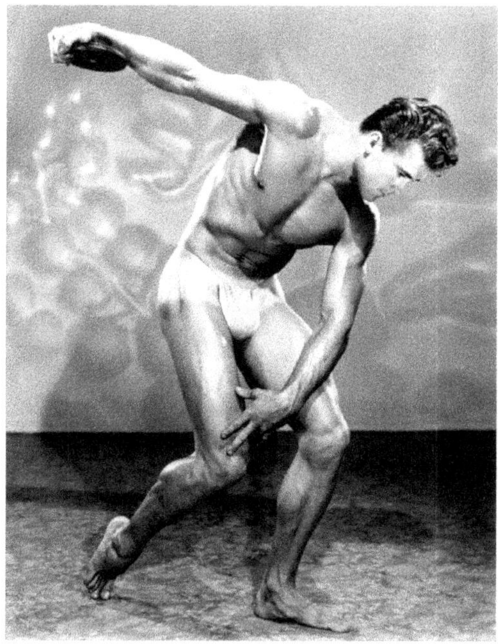

FIGURE 4.9. Ed Fury, physique model, by Bob Mizer (1950s). Courtesy of AthleticModelGuild.com.

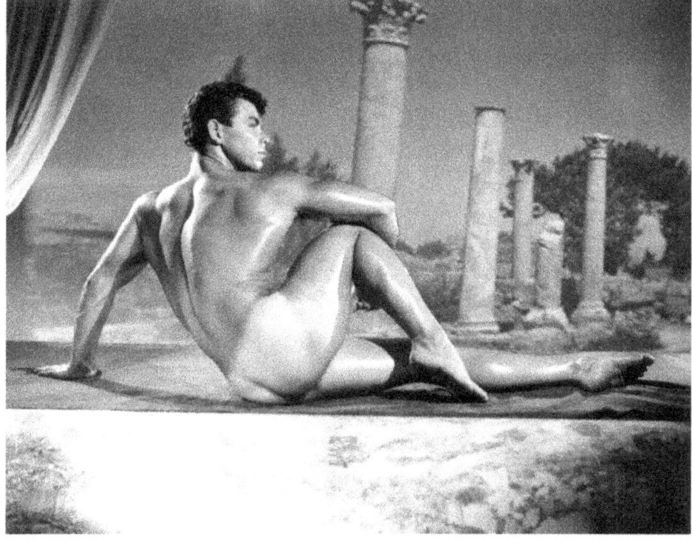

FIGURE 4.10. Unidentified physique model, by Bob Mizer (1950s). Courtesy of AthleticModelGuild.com.

Although the photography of Mizer is largely representative of the muscle boys of his time, it was competitive bodybuilders and women that gave him his initial lens training. Most of Mizer's work was shot at the compound, but Bell reported that where he really got his start was at the famous Muscle Beach, in Venice, California:

> He really started with bodybuilders, those were the models that were trying to get work, so the bodybuilder really lent to that Greek classic ideal. As an aspiring photographer he was shooting everything that he could to pay his rent. He shot a lot of women, a lot of beauty contest as well, which is kind of weird.[14]

Figures 4.11 and 4.12 show some of Mizer's never-before published photographs from this period at Muscle Beach. When I asked Bell what was Mizer's motivation with Muscle Beach, muscle boys, and beefcake, he reported another little-known fact about Mizer:

> Throughout Bob's diaries he's always talking about wanting to work out. He always wanted to be one of these big bodybuilders, but he just couldn't do it, so he found that it was better eventually just to just photograph them. Throughout his diaries, for all the years he kept those, every single day he recorded his weight, every morning and every night.

It was not necessarily talent, but the guts of Mizer that renovated the physique magazines into a gay channel and created the first significant gay mass media. Although the work of Maplethorpe and Lynes can be considered art and that of Mizer's beefcake, we must not undermine Mizer's influence for bringing awareness on a mass scale to what in the 1940s and 1950s was unacceptable and unimaginable: celebrated homosexuality. Not only was *Physique Pictorial* the first magazine dedicated to the body beautiful, it also did not shy

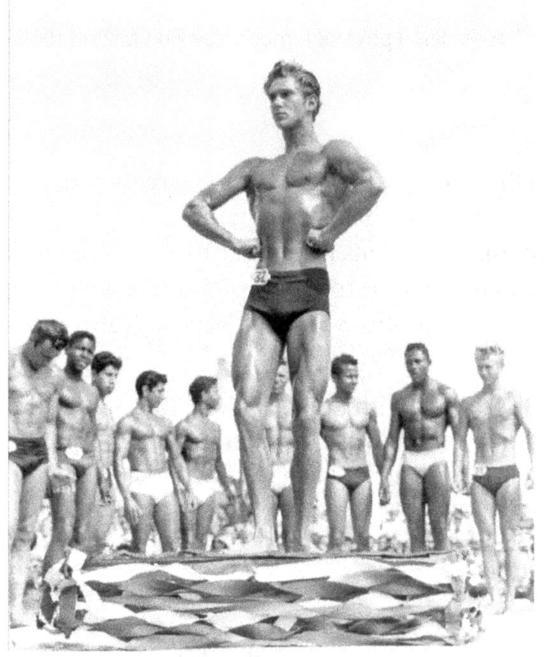

FIGURE 4.11. Unidentified contestant at a Muscle Beach physique competition, by Bob Mizer (1940s). Courtesy of AthleticModelGuild.com.

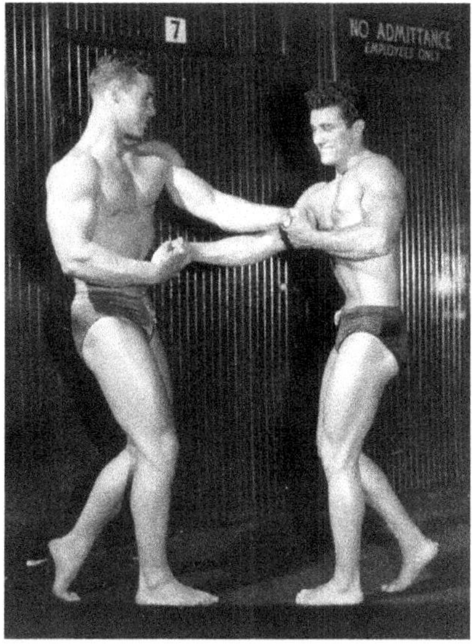

FIGURE 4.12. Unidentified bodybuilders, by Bob Mizer (1940s). Courtesy of AthleticModelGuild.com.

away from its homoerotic content (see Figures 4.13 and 4.14). As Dennis Bell points out:

> If you read the *Physique Pictorials,* at the bottom on many of the pages Bob used to write these lengthy editorials and print them in this tiny, tiny type that you could hardly read. He would argue in favor of controversial issues relating to gay culture and publishing male nudity. Full-frontal nudity was one thing he always wrote about.

The magazine was unapologetically celebrating the male nude and targeted at a gay audience (see Figures 4.15 and 4.16). As F. Valentine Hooven, III, points out in *Beefcake: The Muscle Magazines of America 1950-1970:*

> No serious attempt was made to gloss over the fact that those attractive young men were naked to be looked at and enjoyed. Men, naked for the pleasure of others? That in the fifties, was dangerously radical.[15]

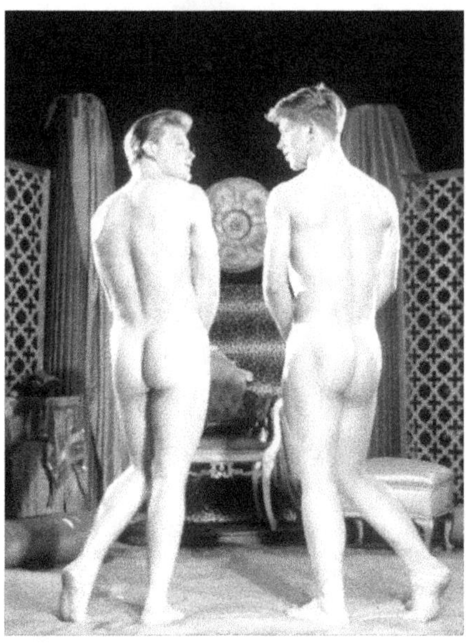

FIGURE 4.13. Bill and Nolan, physique models, by Bob Mizer (1950s). Courtesy of AthleticModelGuild.com.

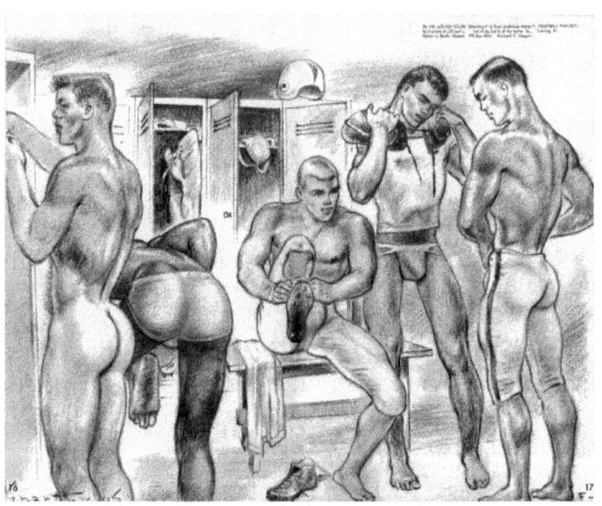

FIGURE 4.14. "In the Locker Room" drawing from Spartacus Series F "Football Practice," featured in *Physique Pictorial,* volume 01, number 09 (1951). Courtesy of AthleticModelGuild.com.

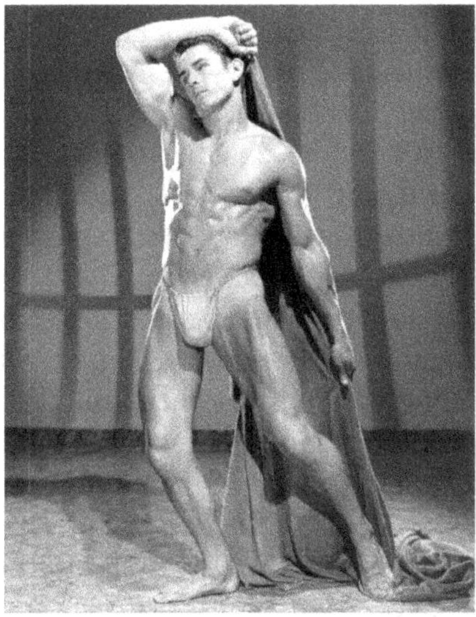

FIGURE 4.15. Leonard Chambers, physique model, by Bob Mizer (1950s). Courtesy of AthleticModelGuild.com.

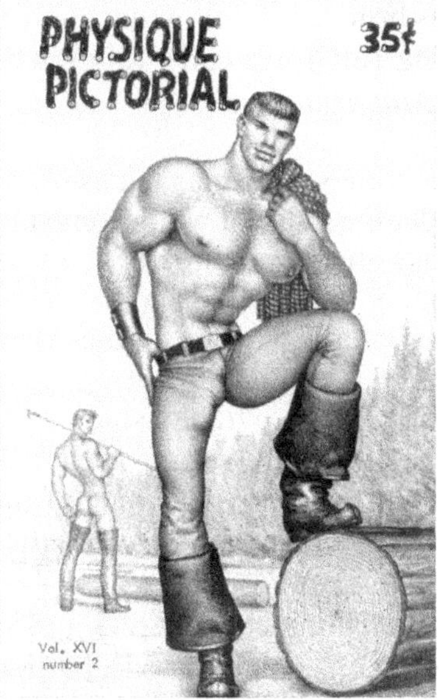

FIGURE 4.16. *Physique Pictorial* cover by Tom of Finland, volume 16, number 2 (1967). Courtesy of AthleticModelGuild.com.

Physique Pictorial was clearly a magazine never attempted before—it was by gay men and for gay men, the first gay magazine and one of the first gay publications. This was a very risky thing to do at the time. Not only was homosexuality outlawed, but the penalties were quite severe, ranging from shock treatment to institutionalization. Censorship and obscenity laws still represented a threat to any gay media, so Mizer was careful to comply with the censors and not show any frontal nudity. The magazine continued to grow and expand its circulation internationally. *Physique Pictorial* was wildly successful, and instigated the creation of other imitation magazines dedicated to the male body beautiful. Among many others were *Adonis, Vin, Grecian Guild, Body Beautiful,* and *Tomorrow's Man.* Hooven estimated that by the 1950s the cluster of physique magazines together reached an annual circulation of one million copies per year sold across the United States and Europe.[16] This *was* the beginning of mass gay media.

The boldness of Mizer and others who followed did not go unnoticed. The criticism and homophobia that Mizer and his comrades came up against was brutal. The following quote is taken from a 1957 article titled: "Let Me Tell You a Fairy Tale," in the then very popular *Strength & Health Magazine.*

> The menace of homosexual magazines is more serious than ever before . . . Under the guise of wholesome physical culture, these dirty little books are aimed directly at a very profitable market, the homosexual or "fairy" trade. What respect can anyone have for a man or boy caught with one of these books in his hands?[17]

Not only were AMG's photography studios at the forefront of gay media, but the magazines were setting the foundation for the next generation of gay men who would integrate the cultivation of the body into their lifestyle, which would eventually give rise to the gay gym.

Mizer died in 1992. Though he was on dialysis the last year of his life, he continued to shoot; according to Bell, Mizer did his last photo shoot a day before he went into the hospital and passed away. In terms of gay media, most scholars agree that Bob Mizer's influence was prettier than a muscle boy picture, as Robert Mainardi told me:[18]

> His influence is huge, not so much having to do with the muscular look, certainly much more to do with a liberating effect of nudity in the 1940s he was taking classical physique pictures as everyone else, but when nudity came in, he went for it gung ho.

Full Frontal

Before full frontal nudity was legally published, there was a huge demand for photographs of nude men, and many photographers had a thriving underground business. These photographers were constantly under the microscope of the authorities. It was not uncommon for their studios to be ransacked by the powers that be and all of their work confiscated and destroyed. After a raid, photographers often closed down their studios and retired from the profession. But the 1960s were a radical time, and extraordinary changes to social structures began to change the attitudes of the people and eventually the laws. Of special interest is a case that ended up in the Supreme Court and involved the shipping of physique magazines catering to a gay audience. The case *Manual Enterprises v. Day* began to change the fate of the physique magazines under scrutiny, and would subsequently have a tremendous effect on gay culture and gay media.

In *Manual Enterprises v. Day,* post office officials had prevented the shipment of the magazines under 18 U.S.C 1461, which barred shipping material that was considered "obscene, lewd, lascivious, indecent, filthy or vile" and made the following claims:

> (1) they were themselves "obscene," and (2) they gave information as to where "obscene" matter could be obtained. The magazines consisted largely of photographs of nude, or nearly nude, male models and gave the name of each model and each photographer and the latter's address. They also contained a number of advertisements by independent photographers offering for sale photographs of nude men.
>
> The Judicial Officer found that the magazines (1) were composed primarily, if not exclusively, for homosexuals and had no literary, scientific or other merit; (2) would appeal to the "prurient interest" of such sexual deviates, but would not have any interest for sexually normal individuals; (3) are read almost

entirely by homosexuals, and possibly a few adolescent males; and (4) would not ordinarily be bought by normal male adults.[19]

To the postmaster's astonishment, the Supreme Court ruled in favor of Manual Enterprises, making the following statement:

> Our own independent examination of [370 U.S. 478, 490] the magazines leads us to conclude that the most that can be said of them is that they are dismally unpleasant, uncouth, and tawdry. But this is not enough to make them "obscene." Divorced from their "prurient interest" appeal to the unfortunate persons whose patronage they were aimed at capturing (a separate issue), these portrayals of the male nude cannot fairly be regarded as more objectionable than many portrayals of the female nude that society tolerates.[20]

The outcome of the *Manual Enterprises v. Day* case had a profound effect on gay culture. Believe it or not, "unpleasant, uncouth, and tawdry" were a step in the right direction. Now that the full nude was accepted, there was very little left to hide. Although it is true that MANual, Trim, and Grecian Guild Pictorial were largely composed of erotic art and their editorial content negligible, they played a substantial role in shaping the gay culture in the decade that would follow. Not only was the male body no longer considered obscene, but with the ruling, homosexuals were given carte blanche to publish and read what they pleased without being prosecuted for material previously considered "obscene, lewd, lascivious, indecent, filthy or vile." This was a *giant* step toward gay organization and liberation.

Following the ruling on *Manual Enterprises v. Day,* other similar legal cases at the Supreme Court level, especially *Miller v. California,*[21] would eventually allow for actual sex to be portrayed in photographs and on film, and a new mega media industry was born: pornography.

PORNOGRAPHY

The beginning of gay pornography would eventually spell the end for the physique magazines. As gay porn became available, the demand for physique magazines diminished dramatically, which confirms that the interest in them was for the most part sexual and not necessarily artistic. The legalization of full frontal nudity was an ironic twist of fate for the physique photography industry, as Dennis Bell told me:

> These people were fighting for this all of these years . . . and once that happened, that frontal nudity was allowed to be published, these same photographers didn't quite know what to do. They didn't know how to handle frontal nudes, and all of them, except AMG, went downhill real fast.[22]

But of course (to use the cliché, when one door closes . . .), Bell continues: "But they did pave the way for studios like Colt and Falcon that really started up big at that time." Gay porn would soon become the most influential media channel for the muscle boy ideal to work its way into gay culture.

The physique magazines of the 1940s and 1950s, and the muscle-clad porn videos and magazines of the 1970s and 1980s were influential in the muscle boy ideal becoming a conventional gay ideal—subsequently establishing and promoting a gay gym subculture. It is well know that men, both gay and straight, buy a lot of porn. Pornography not only explores our fantasies but also is influential in creating new ones. I often joke with my single friends who say they want to be in a relationship that they don't really want a boyfriend, that what they want is a porn star.

If we look at heterosexual pornography of the 1960s and even 1970s, the men are of average build and stature; the focus is predominantly on the women's bodies. But what was appealing to heterosexual men did not work for gay men who basically fantasized about big dicks and even bigger muscles. From the start of commercialized gay pornography, the muscle man was often central to the fantasy. What is interesting is that as pornography worked its way into the mainstream, the leading men of the gay skin flicks worked their way into the straight ones. And of even more interest, the muscle boy ideal worked its way into the minds of the straight male viewers. In the 1980s, there is a noticeable difference in the men who started appearing in heterosexual porn and magazines like *Playgirl*. The biggest difference was the amount of muscle on them. The models and actors of the straight videos now looked just like the muscular models in the gay porn magazines and videos. This is an interesting occurrence, because it is almost exclusively straight men who are viewing straight porn, so if the straight men are viewing the porn for their interest in women, why would the men in the porn need to be muscular? An oversimplified and clearly incomplete answer is that, more likely than not, this has to do with newly adapted ideals of muscularity and masculinity in which men identify or fantasize being the men in the porn, requiring the male porn actors to be beefcake.

Because the change in pornography's body ideals was first seen in gay porn, it is then constructive to examine how this occurred. We could examine changes in gay pornography noting various phases of evolution, but such evolution would be so short lived to suggest that there was not much evolution—because as I have mentioned, beefcake was central to gay pornography from the start. What did evolve, however, was the level of beefcake: the models kept getting bigger and more muscular with every decade. Figures 4.17, 4.18, 4.19, and 4.20 illustrate the hypertrophy of the gay porn star between the 1970s

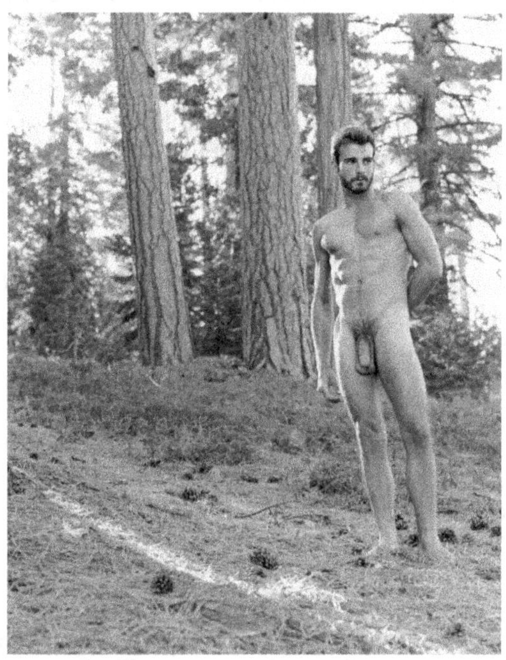

FIGURE 4.17. Al Parker, 1970s porn star and famous "clone," by Jim French (1970s). Courtesy of ColtStudio.com.

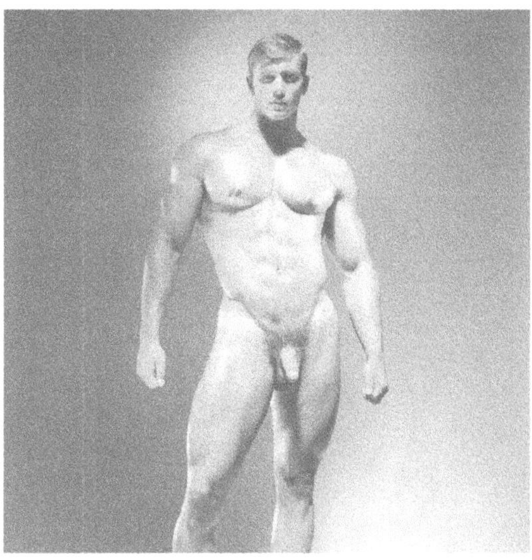

FIGURE 4.18. John Pruitt, porn star, by Jim French (1980s). Courtesy of ColtStudio.com.

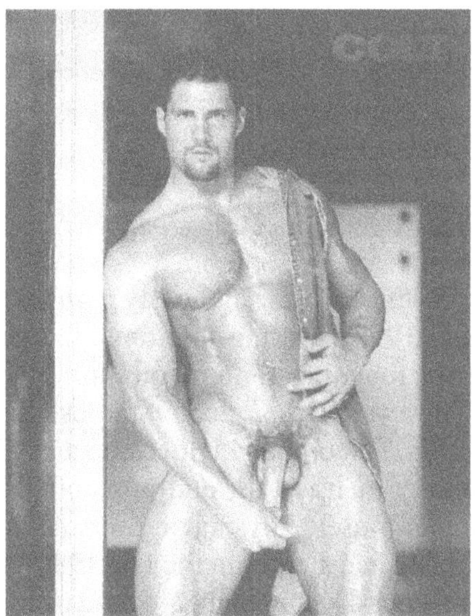

FIGURE 4.19. Franco Corelli, porn star, by Jim French (1990s). Courtesy of ColtStudio.com.

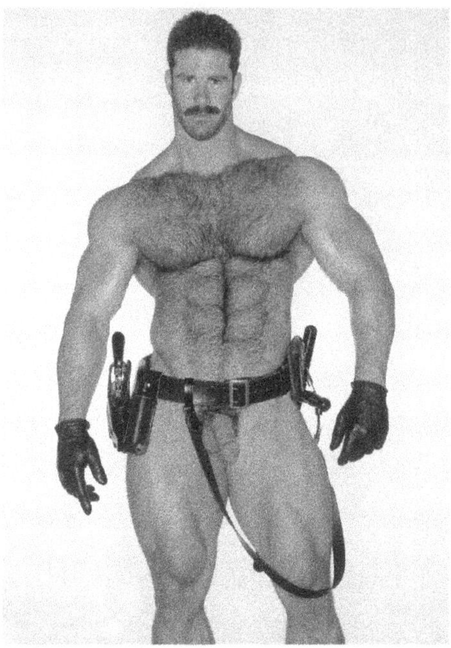

FIGURE 4.20. Pete Kuzak, porn star, by Jim French (2000s). Courtesy of ColtStudio.com.

and the 2000s–clearly demonstrating an approximate twenty pounds of muscle gain per decade, if not more.

The most notable hypertrophy of the gay porn star occurred during the late 1980s and 1990s. During this time, the gay porn industry boomed and saw the founding of numerous porn studios. At the forefront of many, however, was Falcon Studios. Started by Chuck Holmes in the 1970s, Falcon quickly became a gay household word due to the popularity of its films, and probably of most relevance here, the featuring of muscle boys having sex. Although Falcon was already a well-established studio, in the late 1980s a young and avid director, John Rutherford, came on board, and over the course of the next fifteen years he became one of gay pornography's most celebrated directors. He eventually became Falcon's president, and under his direction Falcon ruled the industry for many years. In 2003

Rutherford left Falcon and soon afterward acquired the oldest gay erotica studio of our time, Colt Studio.

Rutherford and I sat down in the conference room of Colt Studio to talk about muscle boys in porn, and specifically about the shift toward a more muscular body image in porn actors during the 1980s and 1990s.[23] "I don't really think it was porn moving in that direction," Rutherford said. "I think it was the community as a whole. Whether you're gay or straight, I think men have become more body conscious over time."

I posed the question: As a director, what has influenced your aesthetic? Rutherford answered:

> Americana, I tend to draw myself towards Alfred Hitchcock or *Thelma and Louise* . . . things that appear normal, clean, and what is acceptable on the outside, but perceived dirty and knotty on the inside. That's my aesthetic, clean packaging but dirty on the inside.

This "Americana" influence is one many of us can relate to, as he told me: "I have to say I'm a TV generation kid, I was raised in front of the TV." In the interest of full disclosure, I should tell you that John Rutherford and I are old friends, we were club kids together, and for several years he was my best friend's roommate. And that is just it—because I have known John as one of the guys, I can tell you that he is as much a product of the American and more specifically, San Franciscan gay culture we grew up in as gay culture is a product of you and me. And this mirroring effect of Americana is what we see in the pornography of John Rutherford as seen in Falcon and Colt, as well as in other modalities of media in general—including my own. Because of this, it is clear to me that the porn of the 1980s and even that of today mirrors what is going on in the subcultures it portrays.

The explosion of muscle-clad pornography was generated by advances in technology. These technological advances are more influential than any specific porn studio, director, or cultural norms. "You have to realize that the film-to-video transition occurred just in 1979," Rutherford stated:

> Everyone used to buy little 8mm film real and you'd have to put up your white screen to sit at home and jack off . . . or before that

> people would go to dark theaters and watch it onscreen, and it was considered very taboo and very dirty.

When video became the medium, he noted, "No more did you need that machine and that white screen."

Another huge technological as well as influential advance in the propagation of porn and muscle media in general is of course the Internet. Even if we do not surf the Internet for porn, distributors of pornography, sex toys, penis enlargement methods, and sex enhancing drugs bombard our computer's mailboxes to the point where we have become almost immune to the material. Whereas a few years ago you would have been shocked or surprised by messages telling you all about "muscle studs, tits, pussy, big cocks, double penetration, and gang bangs," now these messages—and the images they embody—are something you come across on a daily basis, at work, at school, at home, and anywhere you check your e-mail. In this sense, the language and images of porn are more and more becoming a part of daily routines, whether consciously or subconsciously.

We have in fact become so immune and accepting of nakedness and sexuality that the two now assume lead roles in the billion-dollar media empires of fashion and commercial advertising.

FASHION AND ADVERTISING

Pornography is not the only modern medium that has been highly influenced by gay culture. So have the fashion and commercial advertising media industries. In the 1980s, after the muscle boys of the physique magazines became fixtures in the gay ghetto, the muscle boy ideal started to move out of the ghetto and work its way into the rest of the culture. In mainstream media, when naked bodies were present prior to the 1980s, it was naked bodies of women, rarely those of men. The images of muscle boys that would come to be in the mainstream were primarily limited to fitness magazines and gay media. This started to change; by the end of the decade images of muscle boys were common in mainstream media. And as I will explain, gay men are largely responsible for establishing and standardizing images of beefcake into mainstream media and on a mass scale.

Perhaps the most influential moment in fashion and advertising, when the seminude muscle boy became the norm, began with the Calvin Klein underwear campaign launched in 1981. An oversized and striking billboard went up in Times Square with the picture of a muscle boy in nothing but Calvin's white briefs. The campaign was the brainchild of photographer Bruce Weber and stylist Sam Shahid.

In an interview he gave to Tim Adams of *The Observer,* Weber stated that sometimes sexuality is confused with character, and that sex is an action we take, rather than what defines us. Weber further stated that he has had many romances with both men and women.[24] Mr. Shahid, on the other hand, is openly gay. Together, the brawny duo not only staged the most successful underwear campaign ever, but also standardized the homoerotic male nude in mainstream media. After Calvin Klein, Weber and Shahid continued working together for many years and creating just as many shocking but precious moments in advertising, the most significant of which is the racy Abercrombie & Fitch (A&F) catalog.

With the Abercrombie & Fitch catalog, Weber and Shahid pushed the envelope even further than they had with Calvin Klein; it was packed with sexually charged images—both hetero- and homosexual. In many of the catalog's photographs the underwear was playfully pulled down revealing the male model's pubic area or buttocks and in several others the underwear was off completely. Other spreads playfully and erotically portrayed young men playing sports almost naked, hanging out in the locker room, or showering together. Although these scenarios are only suggestive (and it does not get more suggestive than that) in terms of homoeroticism, in a few of the magazines, same-sex couples are shown in romantic embraces. The catalog presented itself more like an artsy magazine packed with beautiful models (verging on soft porn) than a clothes catalog. It quickly became coffee-table matter for urban gay men.

In American commercial advertising, the sexuality of A&F was as risqué as the industry had seen. It was also as successful as it wanted to be: the catalog and images were an overwhelming success, and A&F, which had been for quite some time a tired and dying brand, became the hottest-selling brand among young Americans almost overnight. While young Americans embraced the boldness and imagery of A&F, their elders did not. The catalog was immediately attacked by conservative groups and labeled gay, pornographic, and obscene; déjà vu, yet again, over very similar images to those of the physique magazines. The catalog was so controversial that eventually A&F

started requiring its subscribers to be over age eighteen. Yet its content remained suggestive, graphic, and sexually packed, giving way to more criticism and controversy—so much so that ultimately, the provocative version of the catalog was pulled from the market. Eventually A&F reintroduced the catalog in a very clean-cut and nonerotic version, making it indistinguishable from the average retailer catalog.

The mainstreaming of the muscle boy ideal has had the same mighty effect on the fitness industry, media, and pop culture in general as it did on white briefs—kaboom! Following the Calvin Klein underwear campaign, the jock in white briefs became such a strong image in America that it launched the careers of two of Hollywood's leading men: Tom Cruise in *Risky Business* and Brad Pitt in *Thelma and Louise*. It is now difficult to open a magazine or newspaper, watch a movie, or turn on the TV without half-naked men popping up everywhere in their underwear. The gay soft porn of the recent past has become the standard ideal for modern men, gay or straight.

So the images that were once described as vulgar and offensive are now the same images that are used to market products to males ranging from high school boys to accountants and construction workers—gay or straight. The homoerotic male nude has become the staple image of mainstream media. What is really surprising is not that this was tried, it's that it's worked. The overwhelming success of advertising campaigns like Calvin Klein's underwear ads and Abercrombie and Fitch's racy catalogs and billboards are solid proof that male beauty is more influential and persuasive on heterosexual men than most of them may be comfortable acknowledging.

It is commonplace today to run into young straight men who naively are walking billboards of homoerotic ideals and styling—such as those mainstreamed by media campaigns the like of Calvin Klein and Abercrombie & Fitch. Adding irony to the equation is the fact that, often, these young men might actually be homophobic in the full sense of the word. The popular TV show, *Queer Eye for the Straight Guy,* might be a phenomenon in terms of modern television shows, but in reality, it is a practice much older than television itself.

The line between what's homoerotic and what's not has become so blurred that it is harder to differentiate which advertisements and periodicals are geared toward heterosexual men and which are targeted toward gay men. Current-day fitness magazines for men are a perfect example. I questioned several straight men at the gym on how they feel about the images in these magazines. One of them, "Marc," is a heterosexual, mid-twenties transplant from the Midwest. He loves to work out, and his built physique is quite noticeable even through his work clothes. Flipping through a copy of *Exercise for Men Only* (which he, being a fitness enthusiast, is familiar with and has purchased before), I point to a few of the pictures in the magazine. One shows a model in tight boxer-cut briefs with a noticeable bulge, standing and flexing his whole body as he demonstrates how to use a hand gripper; another page highlights a different jock posing in ripped denim hot pants opened at the fly and showing the pubic area about 2 millimeters above the penis; yet another page depicts a model bending over and suggestively posed to highlight his bubble butt and the V-shaped torso. After pointing out the pictures, I ask Marc what he thinks of the images.

He now goes back and forth between the several pages I pointed to and tells me that he finds the pictures inspiring, in the sense that he "wants to look like that. They motivate me to work out," he adds. When I emphasize the near nudity and suggestive poses, I ask him if he finds the images homoerotic. "Now that I think about it, they kind of are." He proceeds to tell me that he can "see how the images would be attractive to gay men," although he doesn't find them erotic. "I had never really thought about it, I guess," he tells me a little confounded, and I can tell he's being honest. When I show the same images to a female friend, she adds: "It's hard to tell whether it's a straight men's magazine with gay undertones or a gay men's magazine with straight undertones."

Newer modes of media, however, are much more direct.

THE INTERNET: GAYGYMCULTURE.COM

By the 1970s, gay media was in full bloom, and the muscle boy ideal was becoming more and more part of gay culture. In the 1980s not only was the muscle boy ideal at the center of gay media and gay culture, but he had also successfully worked his way into mainstream media. As if this was not enough, the early 1990s saw the invention of the most powerful medium of communication ever conceived: the Internet. In just a few years, the Internet became one of the main channels of information, and the muscle boy ideal then prevalent in gay urban centers worked his way into the screens of gay men around the world.

Gay men in urban, suburban, and rural areas around the globe started to identify with and build themselves into modern-day Apollonian men. In the last decade, the gay muscle boy ideal, classical of Chelsea, the Castro, and West Hollywood, has been globalized via the Internet—it is now a gay global phenomena.

The ideal initially traveled the Internet via advertising, erotica, and pornography. However, as the Internet became a gathering place for gay men, Web addresses increasingly started catering to the building of online communities for men interested in the celebration and cultivation of the gym-built body. Countless Web sites have since been created as places where gay men can chat, share information, admire one another, motivate each other, and probably of most importance, eventually even meet in person.

Of the thousands of Web sites dedicated to the body beautiful in gay culture, bigmuscle.com is one of the most popular. Bigmuscle .com was created and launched by Andy Wysocki and Bill Sanderson. In an exclusive interview for this book, Bill told me about its beginings:[25]

> I'm 6 foot 4, and I see these guys who are 5 foot 5, 5 foot 7—they're always built, and they tend to build muscle a lot quicker. I wanted to build a site where I could see what the characteristics are for building the body of someone who's 6 foot 4 inches. Those were the goals, but one of the underlying goals was that if I build a site and they post the photos I wouldn't have to search the Internet [laughs].

Bigmuscle.com is a Web site where members (membership is free) can post a profile with pictures, geographical location, contact information, and physical statistics (height, weight, chest size, waist size). Each profile features an area where the user can write any text he likes; there's also a section where members can list links to other member profiles on the Web site. But the biggest draws are, without a doubt, the pictures and the unformatted text many of the members write.

Both the pictures and the members' written accounts have turned bigmuscle.com into the hottest online destination for muscle boys and muscle men around the world, and a great number of them have begun calling the Web site a community. This was a surprise even for Andy and Bill, as Andy recalls:[26]

> It grew slowly, but after the first two years, all of a sudden people started telling other people, and that's when it really changed direction. Then people started calling it a community. We never called it a community; I just really looked at it as purely a database to compare stats with. I notice a lot of people will log in just before they go to work to see if they have any messages, and then they log in when they get home.

The pictures posted by members on bigmuscle.com vary from the PG-13 variety of homemade, innocent and funny pictures to artistic nudes and pornographic ones, many taken by professional photographers. All the profiles include pictures of their members' bodies in different stages of undress—from shirtless to full nudes. Sure, you say, the Internet is plastered with images of naked men (and women); however, what makes Web sites like bigmuscle.com different is that, unlike the thousands of other sites where the male nude is commonplace, here the models were not paid to model. They are "regular" guys like you and me who have decided to post their personal and sometimes very intimate pictures and information online for the world to see.

The other winning ingredient to bigmuscle.com is the text the members write. The reasons men post their profiles on Web sites like bigmuscle.com vary greatly—from men wanting to meet friends, dates, and sex partners, to those looking for a life partner or those simply wanting to show off their hard work at the gym or get tips about working out and nutrition. Some profiles do not include any text at all, but the thousands that do vary from the most casual chit-chat about sex, work-out tips, and the weather, to deeply emotional and philosophical conversations about life, athletics, and current events. This type of dialogue is an area that Andy and Bill purposefully encouraged. "We try to make the site more thought driven in making the guys write about themselves," Andy told me. "Granted, there's instant gratification with the photos, but we like to see the profiles where the person writes a long description, because whether you like it or not it tells you a lot about that person."

In my opinion, these self-published, unedited, personal dialogues are what truly add a different, and much more interesting, layer to the muscle boy image in media, because, these accounts—unlike commercial media—connect the image to a real person. A real person who is more than just a pretty picture, and who writes about his plans, goals, and his wants. Bill agrees:

> Getting back to the profiles where people actually write something about themselves to show you that they're just not a body and a photo and there is a person behind that . . . I think having those mini blogs help . . . when you look at one photo, yes that personifies a muscle person, but you know nothing about a photo from a magazine . . . generally with the pin up magazines, it's all written text for marketing . . . its all to embellish the story and the theme. Here they are posting their own information and they are exposing themselves, not only visually but on an educational level, what they're looking for, what they want, and it's making it more personal than just buying that men's magazine and going "oh he's cute," you're getting the real story behind the person and the fact that nine times out of ten you can contact that person and they'll probably contact you back.

Having lived in San Francisco during the dot com boom, I witnessed firsthand countless attempts at creating what bigmuscle.com has done unintentionally: a wildly successful online community. Many of these failed attempts were staffed by an impressive roster of Wharton CEOs, MIT CIOs, and Stanford MBAs all burning millions and millions of dollars disastrously and sometimes ridiculously. On the other hand, I was surprised to learn that Bill and Andy still run bigmuscle.com out of their basement and on their free time while both hold full-time jobs (eight months after our interview Andy finally left his regular job to dedicate full time to running the Web sites). Bigmuscle.com publishes about 21,000 active member profiles, averages 132,000 unique visitors a day, with some days, traffic as high as 140,000—a wet dream in terms of Internet marketing. Yet the success of bigmuscle.com can be explained by a simple marketing-101 concept: it fills a niche. Bill is quick to point out that:

> It kind of surprised us, if you do a search for Bill and Andy you get thousands of people who thank us for building the site and we never thought about that . . . I think it fills a niche, a slice of gay life, and a lot of people, a good percentage of them use it to

communicate with their friends, I think it's just another conduit for people of like mind-sets to hang out together.

The following two e-mails received by Andy and Bill explain how some of bigmuscle.com members feel they are part of a community:

> Andy,
>
> I just wanted to follow up and thank you again for the points to Feature myself. I used them yesterday, and in a word the response was Incred-i-burg-able!!! Over 12,000 views and 200 emails (not that anyone was counting). More importantly, many connections made with some really terrific people. Quite a day, and again quite a forum for such exchanges to occur.
>
> Just wanted you to know how appreciative I am. Hope your weekend is going well . . . mine sure has been a blast! :-)
>
> -Dirk.

Another member writes:

> i'm sure you've been hit by so many kudos that another will seem trivial (in fact, i've already thanked you once for what you've provided.) meaning, this forum, bm.com. i see you've already launched 'normalgay.com' but i have to tell you, that from my experience so far, and i've only been a member since sometime in december, that this community you've created is awe inspiring.
>
> BUT, the compassion, passion, and gentleness that's coming out of some of the profiles, and some of the e-mails I've received from those who find something in 'me' inspiring just makes me . . . pause.
>
> i just ended a 19 year relationship and was unsure as to whether there'd be someone out there for me. i think we all think that when something ends. wishy-washy? nope, just really letting you know that whomever you are, and for whatever reason you're doing what you're doing, i thank you.
>
> have a great day andy.
>
> -john.

Hanging out together is what brings many members to bigmuscle.com. According to Andy:

> A lot of people who work for business and travel write, and they tell us: "I don't have to eat dinner alone anymore," they can now go to city xyz and even if they're not looking for sex, its nice to be able to go meet up somebody and talk and at least know they have the common ground of working out and keeping fit.

From a sociological perspective, online communities like bigmuscle.com have created a media phenomenon: mass-scale, self-published media and erotica. Until just a few years ago, all of the images in media and accompanying text were premeditated, constructed, and promoted by advertisers and directors—used fearlessly to sell their products or films. As you have most likely read in one place or another, social critics have argued (sometimes convincingly) that these images of beauty have been force-fed to the public.

What phenomena such as bigmuscle.com have done is add a layer of complexity to this argument—because bigmuscle.com *is* the public. Today, more men are disrobing and plastering the Internet with their nude or near-nude pictures than commercial media produces. What the thousands and thousands of men who publish their profiles on the Internet every day have done is challenge the argument that we are all victims of Madison Avenue.

MEDIA'S SOCIAL INFLUENCE AND PRESSURE

No discussion of the history, evolution, and standing of muscle media is complete without an analysis of the influence it places on its target audience. A fair and balanced discussion of the influence of the media, keeping our best interests in mind, includes both its positive and negative influence.

In the survey I conducted, respondents were asked whether or not they felt pressured to exercise in order to look good, and if they did, where this pressure came from. The responses varied dramatically on a spectrum ranging from "Not at all pressured" (18.5 percent) to "Extremely pressured" (7.2 percent), with the majority of respondents feeling only "Somewhat pressured" (45.2 percent) (see Figure 4.21).

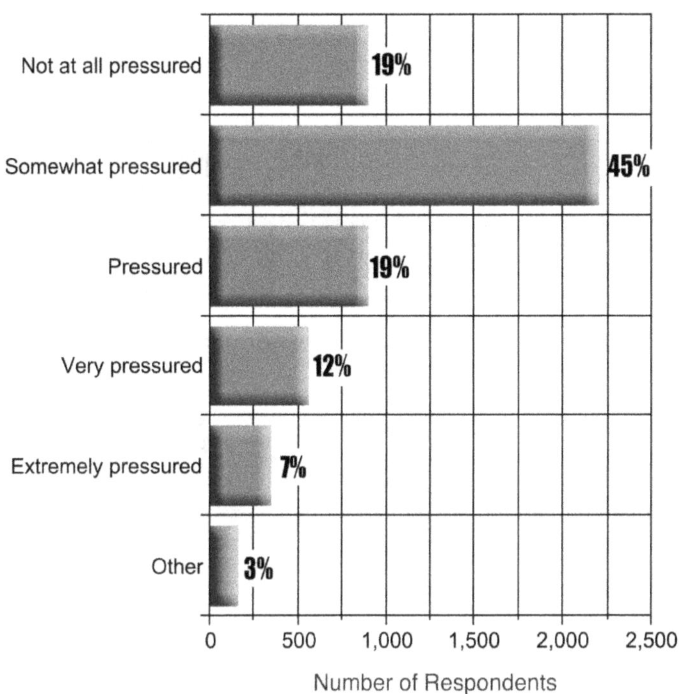

FIGURE 4.21. How much do you feel "pressured" to exercise in order to look good? (multiple answers).

Of those who felt pressured, I asked where the pressure came from. The majority pointed to "Myself" and "Gay culture" as the two primary sources of pressure—sources I will discuss in greater detail in following chapters. Media came up next, specifically print, erotic, entertainment, and online media, which were identified as the third, fourth, fifth, and sixth sources of "pressure," respectively (see Figure 4.22).

Positive Pressure

The positive side of this pressure is the urgency that media instills in men to exercise, eat healthy, and work out. Regular fitness programs provide mental and physical benefits (I will discuss this further in following chapters). When homoerotic representations in media are exercised without censorship, we all, as a community, benefit and

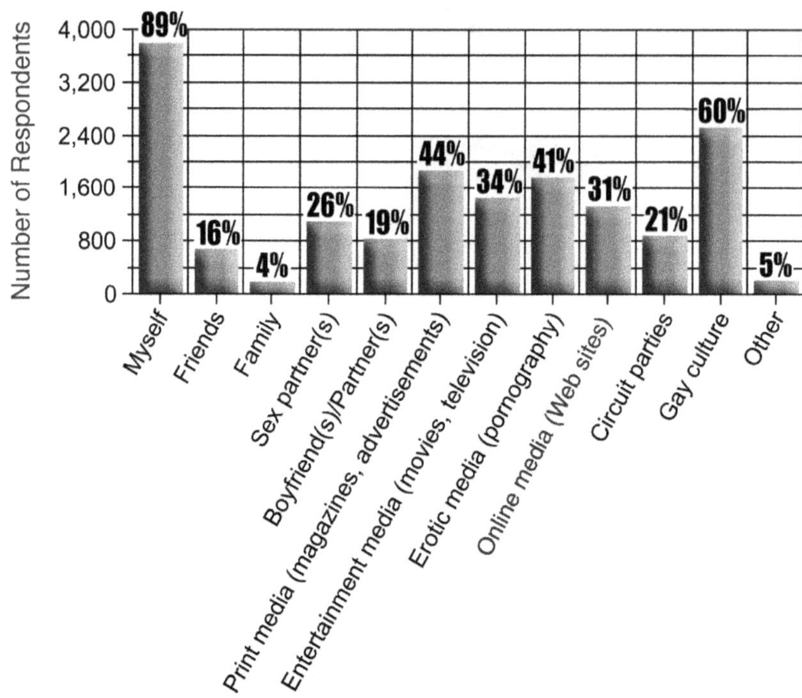

FIGURE 4.22. If you do feel pressured to work out in order to look better, where does this pressure come from? (check all that apply).

advance. When it comes to sexuality, the positive image generated by unrestricted representations of homoeroticism has the potential to give young men the message that they might explore and experience it with less guilt and shame than their gay "fathers" and "grandfathers" ever thought possible.

Negative Pressure

Pressure becomes negative when it generates unhealthy results. Of these, the most dramatic are excessive amounts of stress and a negative self-image. When people feel so much pressure that they feel bad about themselves, we have a problem. This, I believe, can be especially problematic for gay men, who sometimes have low self-esteem in relation to the complexities of being gay, coming out, and living in a predominantly and often intolerant and bigoted straight society. The issue then has the potential to become even more problematic when gay or bisexual men feel this divisive pressure alienating them from gay culture. *Culture*—not media—is the key word here. What I have found is that this type of pressure and alienation, while true and complicated, almost always has more to do with other facets of culture than just media. For example, in the survey I conducted, the hundreds of men who elaborated on why they felt pressured portrayed a more complex world (one we'll discuss more in detail in further chapters), responsible for more pressure than the single word "negative" can describe or define:

> "If I do feel internal pressure I would have to say that it's in part to gay culture as a whole." (twenty-nine-year-old in Toronto, Canada)
>
> "Somewhat pressured by Sexualized society." (thirty-six-year-old, The Netherlands)
>
> "If you want to get laid by a hot dude . . . ya gotta look hot!" (forty-two-year-old in Los Angeles)
>
> "Representing a positive role model in the HIV community." (forty-four-year-old in Washington, DC)
>
> "I get depressed if I go too long without working out. I work out to feel good mentally and physically." (thirty-five-year-old in Houston, Texas)
>
> "Pressured by my physicians—all 3 of them." (forty-year-old, in Fort Worth, Texas)
>
> "My neighborhood: Chelsea."(twenty-five-year-old in New York, New York)
>
> "Except for my health, I'm inspired by many things but not pressured by any of them. Motivated-not pressured. Inspired, not contrived." (forty-two-year-old in Atlanta, Georgia)
>
> "In Psych 101 terms, I am a high self-monitor type. I push myself, for all the right reasons." (forty-eight-year-old Austin, Texas)

The supposedly negative effects of media and negative pressure it is thought to create have been discussed at length (and quite biased) in books such as *The Beauty Myth: How Images of Beauty Are Used Against Women,* and *The Adonis Complex: The Secret Crisis of Male Body Obsession.* These books argue that young men and women today are victims of the beauty-driven mafia, or what they refer to as the media. The authors of these books argue that it is the media that is largely responsible for influencing eating and body image disorders such as anorexia, bulimia, and muscle dysmorphia. As a health professional who has directly worked with people suffering from these disorders, I will be the first to tell you that these problems are not to be taken lightly; they are serious and extremely painful as well as complicated. But I will also tell you that they affect only a tiny percentage of the population, and such numbers simply do not account for the epidemic proportions that the books warn us about.

My research shows that those who feel "extremely pressured," represent the smallest group when compared to those who feel "not at all pressured," and six times less than those who only feel "somewhat pressured." What this means, statistically speaking, is that positive pressure outweighs negative pressure by 93 percent.

The downfall of researchers and social critics, when discussing eating and body image disorders and identifying the media as their cause, is the fact that these problems are complicated and multidimensional. Rarely, if ever, are the roots of low self-esteem and negative self-image directly proportional to just one topic. Images in media might reinforce and even fortify the problem, true, but more likely than not, these images did not create it wholly. Nor has the media the potential to solve them.

Another interesting point is that although the muscle boy ideal dominates male image in mainstream media, countless sources are celebrating other body types—from the skinny-twink variety to the chub-and-round, and everything else in between. Bigmuscle.com was so successful that Andy and Bill later started bigmusclebear .com, which has been just as successful and currently publishes 19,000 active member profiles and receives 61,000 unique visitors a day. Bigmusclebear.com celebrates the "muscle bear" ideal. In fact, Bill and Andy tell me that they often receive requests from members of bigmuscle.com to take their profiles down because they have posted one on bigmusclebear.com where they feel more comfortable.

Most recently, Andy and Bill started normalgay.com as an answer to the many requests they received for a nonbody-specific online community. Clearly, body ideals are diversifying—the dialogue is changing—and this will, no doubt, have an unprecedented, yet undetermined, domino effect on pop culture and more specifically male body image, not to mention the media that complies with demand.

An interesting point from a media perspective is that the demand is quite easy to supply. Porn powerhouse Colt receives 30 to 100 submissions from potential models every week; Falcon receives even more. Yet this is more models than Colt can potentially use. According to Rutherford: "we literally have to tell models, 'I'm sorry, we really want to work with you, but we don't have anything going on right now, so stay tuned.'"[27] Furthermore, as much authority as "big and built" have in pornography today, there are signs that "supersize" is not everybody's Happy Meal. Dennis Bell told me that there is an increasing demand for physique photography similar to that from Mizer's era:[28]

> I think there's been a little bit of a change back to the natural build again. People are tired of the shaved, prepped, guy full of makeup, that whole look. This also lends itself to a lot of the stuff that's going on the Web right now, all the amateur sites, the amateur cam and live video . . . the just see it as it is.

Advertising and media is nothing more than a chain of supply and demand. The public has not only been receptive to such images, the public increasingly demands them. Do these images affect and influence us? Absolutely. Do we as a public accept and demand them? No question about it.

In this chapter I have discussed the historical events that have led to where we are today in terms of body image, body culture, and media; it did not just happen all of a sudden. These cultural norms evolved from a series of different factors, not a single one that we can just ignore or change as some social critics with limited attention spans or historical knowledge have suggested. It is not just media, or porn, or nudity, or the gym, or the Gay Movement, or the Sexual Revolution, or the Women's Movement, or television, or the movies, or the Internet, or the printing press, or the photograph, or strongmen. It is all of these factors involved.

Think about gym-built bodies and the many forms of media that represent them. The male homoerotic body is objectified and commercialized in every possible way. At the same time, it is celebrated. This is a true catch-22—because objectification and commercialization cannot possibly occur without social approval and desirability. When the homoerotic body was concealed and censored, so was homosexuality. There is an important level of politics attached to the free expression of homoeroticism in media.

THE GAY IDEAL

The gay muscle boy ideal is fast becoming the mainstream male ideal. This is an interesting trend, because while for gay men, the ideal makes sense in that it is based largely on our sexuality—we pursue what we're attracted to—the mechanism is a little different for straight men and really not as reasonable. In terms of media and male image, the ideal image of modern heterosexual man is by and large built on the fantasies of gay men, not those of women. A hard, naked, muscular body does not, for the most part, rank high on the desirability spectrum for attracting women, but it does for gay men. From the time of the Greeks and likely before then, it always has. A perfect modern example is the failure of *Playgirl* to attract female readers. Even though *Playgirl* is the only magazine of its type catering to heterosexual women, a very large percentage of its subscribers are men.

Although the most dramatic changes in modern gay culture have occurred since the onset of gay liberation in the 1970s, the ideal gay man had been developing for decades before Stonewall. This process of challenging old stereotypes has not been completed, and it is impossible to predict just how much more change will occur or possibly how much we'll regress. But we could safely assume that when it comes to issues of sexuality and male image, this is only the edge of the vortex.

In the past 100 hundred years, 2,000-year-old stereotypes have been challenged so much that while the mold of old stereotypes is not shattered, they are no longer tangible. Culturally speaking this is how gay culture is affecting and changing Western history. It is certainly no coincidence that male nudity and homosexuality continue to surface and peak at similar times in history. If we look at the most influential men in the creation of the current male physique ideal from the

Renaissance to the twenty-first century, the list is for the most part made up of homosexual and bisexual men, with a few token heterosexual men, whose heterosexuality has been not just questionable, but in many cases—ambiguous. If the Renaissance period saw a revival of the classical in art, architecture, and literature, the nineteenth century saw a true renaissance in the practice of cultivating the body beautiful. As we will discuss in the following chapter, gay men gave renaissance to a new version of the homosexually charged Greek gymnasium.

Chapter 5

The Gay Gym

At one of the most popular gay gyms in San Francisco, the crowd is pumping. It is a Monday evening, and hundreds of gay men, mostly in their twenties, thirties, and forties work their bodies to the beat drumming on the sound system or their iPods. During prime gym time (4 to 8 p.m.) if you were to dim the lights, the scene would resemble a busy nightclub—minus the cocktails. This is one of the most popular, largest, and most diverse gyms in San Francisco; it is home base to a mixture of muscle boys, circuit boys, muscle bears, athletes, poz jocks, and older males. The place draws the prettiest boys, the hottest men, and the buffest bears in the city.

Friends or boyfriends meet after work and work out together, and others can count on running into their friends here. For many, the gym is only part of their social life, but for others it is their only interaction with the gay social world. Testosterone is in the air, and so is sex. Besides lifting and pulling on iron, some men are involved in deeply intellectual or emotional conversations; others chat casually, flirt, and some even try to block out all that is going on and get a good workout. In fact, this gym can at times be such an intense social scene that many gay men prefer to go somewhere else, while others keep a membership there for when they are in the mood to be in such an environment, which they describe as akin to "going out." Most recently, during Gay Pride week, the gym and a popular local nightclub collaborated, and for one night the muscle boys worked out to a well-known DJ (disc jockey) spinning records at the gym. At times like this, the line between social club and health club blurs almost completely.

In large gay ghettos such as San Francisco, New York, Fort Lauderdale, and Los Angeles, gyms like this are a rapidly growing social outlet for thousands of gay men. In these large gay enclaves, the gym has, for a great number of gay men, completely replaced Happy Hours

Muscle Boys: Gay Gym Culture
Published by The Haworth Press, Taylor & Francis Group, 2008.
doi:10.1300/6034_05

at the bars that were so popular in gay culture during the 1970s and 1980s. In fact, between the hours of 4 and 8 p.m. in San Francisco, the gay gyms are much busier than any of the local gay bars. In large urban centers the gay gym has become for many gay men the new Happy Hour.

In this chapter I will discuss the history and rise of the gay gym in gay ghettos as a result of the gay liberation and organization movement. I will focus on how the gym went from being an obscure social institution to becoming one of the most important social centers in gay culture today. Then, I will look at how the gay gym started changing, shaping, and influencing gay culture—both physiologically and socially. Finally, I will discuss how the gay gym continues to emerge as a dominant and influential subculture within gay society.

GAY LIBERATION AND THE RISE OF THE GAY GYM

Gay liberation was about many things. It was about expressing our homosexuality without the shame or fear that had been attached to it for so long. It was about claiming civil rights that had been denied to homosexuals for much of the previous 2,000 years in Western culture. It was not just about expressing and accepting our sexuality, but celebrating it. And in the case of the gay gym and the male body it was about reclaiming the male physique as our own and at the same time demystifying the homosexual body.

When Cecil Franco (a pseudonym), a seventy-nine-year-old man, who was gay before we started using the word "gay," first walked into a popular gay gym in San Francisco a few years ago, he was shocked at how muscular and masculine the men where. Cecil tells me that: "I had no idea gay men could look like that; when I was younger the only way for men to be gay was to be sissies."

When I mention Cecil's reaction to Brendan Eaton (a pseudonym), a gay twenty-two-year-old Berkeley college student, he seems surprised and curiously asks: "Really? I thought gay men always looked like that." He continues to tell me that he has basically assumed that "having a muscular body and being masculine is just part of being gay."

What is interesting about the polarity of the statements given by Cecil and Brendan is that each one is correct, given the times and environments they have lived in. What a difference a generation makes.

In the next few chapters I will discuss in much more detail how masculinity is a social construction that gay (like straight) men have learned to manipulate; but for the meantime, let's discuss masculinity on two of its most basic levels: how it is displayed and how it is perceived.

Before gay liberation, gay men who were masculine concealed their homosexuality. Only those who were, or appeared, somewhat feminine were perceived as gay. The former, culturally speaking, were invisible and the latter were seen as abnormal and deviant and were largely rejected by the main establishment. Labeled *sissies,* the effeminate homosexual represented all homosexuals for centuries in Western culture. Before Stonewall, among gay circles, the masculine gay men were not completely absent but were also not completely visible. Referred to as "butch," or "butches," they were somewhat visible but as a whole not representative of the subculture. Back then, even other gay men perceived the "butch" gay man as an anomaly. Prior to the 1960s and 1970s, the consensus was that all homosexual men were frail, weak, effeminate, and limp-wristed. The notion that a man could be both homosexual and masculine was not even entertained. The 1970s, of course, changed all this: men from all walks of life and all points on the masculinity spectrum started coming out and acknowledging their homosexuality in public. The image of gay men started to change.

Many of the early pioneers of gay culture contested the "sissy" stereotype: gay men were now just like other men and were present in every position and career track: cops, firemen, and lawyers, to accountants, bus drivers, and construction workers.

Of course, gay liberation was also about accepting our femininity as much as it was about reclaiming our masculinity. Now we had the option. At the gay ghettos, we could be glamour drag queens or we could be construction workers, or we could be both. In fact, during the beginning of the gay ghetto, much of gay culture revolved around the exploration of gender bending (a practice that we can still observe quite often in young gay men and lesbians coming to terms with and exploring homosexuality). The gay ghettos quickly became expressions of both hyperfemininity and hypermasculinity. Although the hyperfeminine gay male stereotype had been exhausted, a new form in the way of hypermasculinity gave way to new ideals in body image and masculinity—muscles were added to the equation of being gay and the muscle boy ideal, prevalent today, started gaining popularity.

In the past, a gay man who appeared and behaved masculine could go to a gym as long as he concealed his homosexuality. If he did not stay in the closet, the situation could even be dangerous. This meant that gay men could fantasize and even photograph and distribute muscle boy media in private, but becoming muscle boys themselves was not really a viable option for many. This changed when gay men in the Castro district of San Francisco, West Hollywood, and the Village in Manhattan started opening their own gyms.

The Gay Gym

It is difficult to pinpoint exactly when and where the first modern gay gyms opened. Partly, this is because most of these places are now closed or have been absorbed by larger and mainstream corporations. But historians have also failed to tell their story: because the separation in the academic mind between brains and brawn lingers, most gay historical societies have not kept records of the gay gyms in the same way that the bars, bathhouses, and even coffee shops and other gay meeting places have been chronicled.

Through interviews with older gay men and research of old gay publications in which the gyms were advertised, I have learned of a few of the first gay gyms that preceded my generation and have since disappeared.

In New York City, the first identifiable gay gym was the Sheridan Square Gym, which opened in the 1960s in the heart of the West Village (fewer references also mention the YMCA on east 48th Street). The Chelsea Gym superceded Sheridan Square Gym in the early 1980s and the new Ironhouse enjoyed several years of being the gym of choice for gay Manhattanites. In the late 1980s and early 1990s, places such as the David Barton Gym, New York Sports Club, Crunch, and Chelsea Piers moved into the gay neighborhoods of New York City and took over.

Michael Meehan, a retired public school official who started working out in January of 1966, used to take three trains from Brooklyn into Manhattan to go work out at Sheridan Square Gym. "There weren't many gyms around," Meehan noted. But even when there were, they were not gay friendly. Even places like Sheridan Square Gym, Meehan tells me, kept a low profile:[1]

> It was New York City in the 1960s, and any place that would serve a drink to three homosexuals together was questioned. So although Sheridan Square Gym may have had a large percentage of gay people, it was not discussed.

San Francisco's first gay gyms were Solarius and Apollo, which operated during the 1970s in San Francisco's first gay neighborhood surrounding Polk Street. When the gays started moving to the Castro District in the 1970s, places in that neighborhood like Muscle Systems, The Pump Room, City Gym, and Market Street Gym took over the stage. The Pump Room later became the "Women's Gym," a women-only gym that catered largely to lesbians, and then a personal training studio. In the Castro district, Market Street Gym was the most popular of all gay gyms, but it was sold in 2002 to Gold's Gym. Of the original gay gyms in San Francisco, Muscle Systems survived the longest until it was sold in 2004 and changed names to "Gym SF." (The last of the original three owners had died of AIDS a few years back and Muscle Systems was inherited by his young and straight male nephew in New York who sold the gym in 2004 to gay owners.) All of the original gay gyms in San Francisco are now gone. The most popular gyms with large numbers of gay-held memberships today are the two Gold's Gyms (south of Market and Market Street), followed by World's Gym (Potrero) and Crunch (Van Ness), both of which are not considered gay gyms per se, but cater to a very mixed and large gay clientele.

In Los Angeles, an all-male gym by the name of Eastons on Beverly Boulevard apparently was the dominant gay gym during much of the 1970s. Eastons was followed by the Sports Connection on Santa Monica Boulevard in West Hollywood. Sports Connection was the gym of choice for gay West Hollywood during much of the 1980s and the earlier part of the 1990s. Today, Gold's Gym and Crunch in West Hollywood are two of the most popular gyms for gay men and gay gym culture in the City of Angels.

Meehan, who also lived in Los Angeles during the 1970s before moving to San Francisco, remembers the crowd at Easton's being largely gay and made up of people in show business:[2]

> Bob Mackey [Cher's costume designer] was there all the time. It was really a lot of guys in show business in one aspect or another . . . that was right before actors started to work out, if you look at movies from the era, if actors like Paul Newman or Robert Redford had their shirts off their bodies were slender . . . very slender bodies were in then, not big and buff like today.

Although we might never really know the details about the first gay gyms, we do know that in the 1970s the gay gyms started becoming social centers for gay men; at the same time they also started influencing gay culture and literally transforming the image of gay men. The change was both physical and cultural. As gay men were redefining homosexuality and masculinity, the gay gyms played a crucial role in redefining the new gay male image. Physically, the new version of the gay muscular male began shattering the mistaken notion that all homosexuals were effeminate, frail, and weak. Culturally, the diversity of gay men began educating the world that homosexuals come in every conceivable ethnotype.

Several things were happening simultaneously that explain the allure of the gym for the gay men of 1970s. For the first time in modern history, large groups of gay men were coming together and organizing; these men were about being who they were, and the gamut ran from the most feminine to most masculine. On one end of the spectrum, drag and its "Court system of Queens" was in full bloom; on the other end, gay men started embracing and displaying overt masculinity—a display which, at least visually, can be asserted by bulging muscles.

As gay men started reclaiming their masculinity and the male physique as their own, the idea of the sissy gay man started to change. Muscles, synonymous with masculinity, went hand in hand with idealized masculinity. The homoeroticism of the physique magazines was brought to life. Gay liberation supported the argument that gay and masculine could be synonymous. As in everything else, gay men wanted to prove that they, too, could do it just as well as straight men, and sometimes better. And building their muscles was, at the very best, effective and visual proof; at the very least, it was a solid argument.

It should be noted, however, that the gender-bending elements of camp and drag were also a part of the popular gay gyms of the 1970s and 1980s. During this time the most common jargon used by gay men to define themselves or other gay men who worked out were *gym queen* or *muscle queen*. These terms are still used frequently today, albeit more often by older gay men. In addition, gay gyms like the old Muscle Systems in San Francisco were affectionately better known as "Muscle Sisters." In fact, before the gym was sold, during Halloween every year, this gym, full of butch men, would hold one of the biggest and most popular drag competitions in San Francisco. The Muscle Sisters contest was famous for the buffest and most muscular drag queens anybody had ever seen.

Drag was wildly popular in the gay ghettos during the 1970s, but there was also a popular and even more influential look and mode of dress and style: the *clone*.

THE CLONE

The in-your-face masculinity of the early gay ghettos was portrayed and displayed by the well-known *clones*. Clones were gay men who adopted a uniformed mode of dress made up of tight Levi 501s, black leather boots, and fitted muscle T-shirts; the look was further masculinized by facial hair—always a moustache and sometimes a beard. Ruggedly handsome, butch acting, the clone was not only the opposite of the sissy, he quickly became the gay male aesthetic ideal of the 1970s. The clone represented the first official gay muscle man known to modern culture. He was the embodiment of the bikers, "rough trade," and athletes whose images graced the pages of *Physique Pictorial* and other gay physique magazines. Porn star Al Parker (Figure 4.18) was one of the most famous clones of his time. He was the gay muscle boy ideal come to life. Even today, it is not uncommon to hear older gay men and lesbians refer to modern muscle boys (such as athletes, circuit boys, and muscle bears) as clones in direct reference to the 1970s archetype.

Historians have often related the clone to the art of Tom of Finland (see Figure 4.9). In many aspects, we find elements of Tom's men in the image of the clone. This, I believe, is only part of the puzzle. While the clone was always a representation of hyper-masculinity, muscles sometimes were and other times were not part of the picture. One of the biggest myths about the clone is that he was always muscular. This is just not true. Some clones were in fact muscular, but others were not at all. Back in the 1970s muscles were not an essential ingredient of the idealized clone aesthetic. Yet Tom of Finland's art depicted only muscular men. It was, however, those clones who were muscular who started popularizing the muscle boy ideal, but it was just the beginning. In an account of life imitating art, although the art of Tom of Finland was nevertheless influential, it was only influential to a limited extent.

I have often read negative references toward the clone for his lack of originality, and mass mentality. Modern critics seem to forget that these young men were more than just fashion victims. In 1971 it took great courage, not to mention great risk, to be a part of the Gay Revolution that has made it so comfortable and safe for gay men today to freely be who they are. By dressing and looking the part, Mr. Clone was publicly proclaiming his homosexuality—a strong political statement even by today's standards. When we look at the clone from a sociological and historical point of view, the very concept was not just original but groundbreaking for the 1960s and 1970s. If we think in terms of the times the clones lived in, we realize that they were, by and large, the gay movement. Although on the surface and at the most simple level the clone represented a physical and aesthetic ideal, they were true revolutionaries beyond the confines of superficiality.

During the 1970s, gay men's interest in developing their bodies was part of the social revolution that was taking place in challenging the gay stereotype. Robert Mainardi remembers that:[3]

> As gay culture developed and gay men began to discover that there were so many other gay men, I think—not on a conscious level but on some sociological level—they developed this desire to develop a gay image for men that wasn't a flaming queen, which is about the only other stereotype there was. This was a period when gay men didn't mind being labeled. They wanted to say "I'm a gay man." To make people notice it, you'd have to have some sort of an image, and I think Tom of Finland and Jim French and other influences pushed this look that became the gay look. Eventually it mutated into the more muscular man.

The clone was the first of many modern times gay ideals. But the clone was also the embodiment of gay men reclaiming those things that society had denied homosexual men for centuries: their body, their masculinity, and, ultimately, their manhood.

The clone has in fact generated both controversy and admiration. But regardless of how you perceive the famous honcho, you cannot ignore the influence that the group's image as a whole had in the mainstream's perception of male homosexuals. In the public's view, the sissies started being perceived as hypermasculine—being a gay man went from being a sissy to being a "sansome." We broke one stereotype with another one—a process that continues today, albeit with different modern stereotypes (e.g., bears, circuit boys, etc.). And this, no doubt, continues to have a domino effect on gay men and gay culture as well as the way in which others perceive us. The clones started a trend with the gay gym that is going strong long after they themselves disappeared almost completely from the Castro, Santa Monica Boulevard, and Christopher Street.

If we take a hard look, the defining characteristics of the clone are not completely absent from gay culture, even though the AIDS epidemic did away with almost their entire generation. Rather, the trend has evolved into the masculine gay subcultures of today, especially the leather and bear communities as well as circuit culture.

THE PUBLIC HOMOEROTIC BODY

Before gay liberation, gay men often met one another for sex in public places such as city bathrooms and highway rest stops. The risk of getting caught was reason for them to keep some, if not all, of their clothes on rather than being completely nude. After liberation, bars and bathhouses quickly became the main meeting places for gay men, and at these places the body started being stripped and displayed. Nakedness, much as it was at pagan festivals of the ancient past, increasingly became part of the celebration. The bodies of gay men went from concealed to stripped. For the previously repressed and oppressed gay man, *naked* quickly became the new black.

The bathhouses in big cities doubled as media outlets, where body ideals became celebrated, pursued, and passed on. As Mainardi remembers:[4]

> Body image developing in the baths? Absolutely. This was also the period when gay media developed. There were little give away papers and newsletters of all kinds that often had model

> ads in the back of them, and those periodicals got distributed to the hinter lands. That influenced people who weren't in the cities, who weren't as exposed to the body culture. They could finally open these papers and see pictures of guys and what they looked like and what the popular image was.

At the bathhouses, gay men were typically nude or covered only by a towel. The naked male body, among homosexuals, started assuming, in real time, a premium it had not seen since the time of the ancient Greeks. Now that they could freely look at naked bodies, the preference was for nice ripped ones, not flabby and unappealing ones. The body started becoming the currency of gay culture, and the muscular and gym-built body quickly became its Ben Franklin. The muscular gym-built body starting being idealized, and the new gay gyms provided both an option and a tool for gay men who wanted to compete in the new gay market.

In fact, the bathhouses were some of the first public places to offer the use of a gym to gay men. Of course, the small gyms at the bathhouses were very much used as props in connection with the homoeroticism associated with the gym, and they doubled as play spaces where men could both work out and have sex—and more often than not, the workout was skipped in order to get to the sex. The historical connection between the traditional gym and traditional gay bathhouses is a discussion I examine in more detail in the locker room chapter (Chapter 12).

During the 1960s and up until the 1980s, when most of the bathhouses closed, bathhouses often commissioned original artwork and murals to be used as decoration and advertising. Bathhouse art was charged with two elements: sex and muscles. There is no question that this art was influential in the building and rising popularity of gay gym culture. Given the circumstances under which this artwork was viewed (during, right before, or after sex), it makes sense that it would have more of an impact and be of greater influence than other media outlets.

In the 1970s the gym and the gym-built body started becoming, for gay men, associated with mating and sex, and this is the reason the subculture has grown so much and become so influential. For better or for worse, the association between the gym and mating, as I will discuss in the next few chapters, is one that continues to be a prevailing force today.

THE GAY GYM TODAY

Gay gyms have evolved into cultural points for many gay men in most of the gay ghettos. Cities like San Francisco, New York, and Los Angeles are now host to not just one but often several gyms that cater primarily to gay men.

Today, gay gym culture pioneers like Michael Meehan marvel at how open and free gay gyms are in comparison to the recent past:[5]

> In the 1960s you wouldn't see guys touching each other in an affectionate way at all. I don't think I saw it in the seventies either. Now, at Gold's Gym [in San Francisco], I see it all the time.

Meehan brings up the name of a well-known, high-ranking public official in San Francisco whom he sees at his gym almost every afternoon. His eyes open wide as he tells me:

> I saw him working out with someone the other afternoon, and the way he was holding the guy and looking in the guy's eyes, and touching him, I thought . . . "They're not just workout partners!" You wouldn't have seen that years ago, you wouldn't have seen that at all.

Gay gyms have evolved from small gyms that were independently owned and not often well equipped, to corporate-owned megagyms that house—literally—tons of the latest equipment. This happened for several reasons: For one, the AIDS epidemic wiped out much of the initial group of gay gym culture, including many gay gym owners, resulting in both the emotional and financial bankruptcy of the gyms and countless other gay establishments and institutions. Second, the assimilation of gay culture in the 1980s welcomed corporate America into the gay ghettos, and fitness conglomerates were quick to jump onboard. Third, the tipping point of fitness and body culture was occurring in America during the same decade, so supply and demand fueled the competition. Large fitness conglomerates such as Gold's Gym, Crunch, and the New York Sports Club have opened or acquired gyms in gay neighborhoods and actively pursue the gay client. In the new tradition of corporate America, some of these organizations directly market, and advertise to gay men. In addition, they sponsor and support gay causes, benefits, and celebrations such as gay pride events, circuit parties, and street fairs. The friendliness toward gays was not always there, however. In San Francisco for example, owners of some of the larger and now heavily gay-attended gyms were initially unenthusiastic and opposed to the large influx of gay clientele at their gyms. These feelings swiftly and quietly changed, however, as the new gay clients purchased gym memberships and other services by the thousands, rapidly exceeding the heterosexual entrepreneur's profit expectations. The same previously homophobic gym owners nowadays go out of their way to lure the gay male client—going as far as spending thousands of dollars to decorate the gym during gay pride week and lavishly spending on award-winning floats for the gay pride parade.

Mainstream and corporate-owned gyms pursuing the gay market is a result of modern economics. The power of the gay dollar has never been clearer. As one of the managers of a popular gay gym in San Francisco recently told me:[6]

> Gay men are more serious about fitness and aesthetics; they have a higher disposable income and are willing to spend more money on personal training, supplements, and tanning.

From a business standpoint, it makes complete sense to pursue the gay male client. "There was no question in my mind that if I wanted to be a successful personal trainer in San Francisco, I should cater to gay men," says former San Francisco trainer Eric Friedman, who is straight.[7] "The amount of clients one can have quadruples at a gay gym." Eric is correct: There is a noticeable difference in the volume of personal training between mostly gay and mostly straight gyms in metropolitan areas. This niche has become wildly profitable for the personal training industry. Given the high disposable income of many urban gay men, the concerns for maintaining health and beauty well into our golden years, and the active sex lives of gay men in the most extraordinary meat market that is the gay world, the gay male client is truly the personal trainer's dream client. So much so, that in cities like New York, Los Angeles, and San Francisco, an increasing number of personal trainers—most of them straight males—have zeroed in on gay men as their target clientele.

The influx of corporate America into the gay gym market has resulted in several dramatic changes within the dynamics of gym culture. To start with, a major impact was the transformation of the gay gyms from men-only spaces into coed ones. Probably the most important effect has been patrons' dress: the gyms have been given a more conservative and clean-cut image. The old gay gyms encouraged partial nudity: men often worked out shirtless, wearing just a pair of shorts and athletic shoes. There are many accounts of men, back in the 1970s, who would work out in nothing but a jockstrap. And at least at one gym, Mainardi remembers, even the jockstrap was optional:[8]

> The first gym I ever joined was called the Apollo gym, in the Tenderloin, in 1971 or 1972. It was specifically a gay gym and a nude gym: you could work out in the nude. The guy who ran it was named John Adams, and he had done some modeling. He really based it on the Greek ideal. There was certainly a sexual atmosphere, but it was just a regular old gym, and I would say half of the people who went worked out in the nude. It was a kind of amateurish bodybuilding atmosphere.

In direct contrast, modern gay gyms have dress codes, and going shirtless is simply not allowed (some more conservative and definitely heterosexual-oriented gyms do not even allow tank tops or very short shorts). The dress code enforced by newer corporate gyms was initially greeted with contempt by many gay men who were used to working out shirtless or simply enjoyed watching those who were. But they had few options. And those gay men who spend quite a bit of time at the gym, have, for the most part, accepted the changes along with the upgrades. Not because they prefer dress codes, but because the conglomerates often offer better facilities and equipment and sometimes longer hours.

The small, individually owned gay gyms of the gay ghetto, where gay gym culture first bloomed, have been, for the most part, absorbed by the mainstream, medium-to-large corporations. A once-obscure gay gym culture blossomed into the powerhouse that it is today. A few small, primarily gay gyms remain scattered around the country in places like San Francisco, Palm Springs, and Fort Lauderdale, but they now serve only a fraction of gay gym culture.

Even today, one of the differences between predominantly gay and predominantly straight gyms is how much skin the members bare. At the more gay-populated gyms, short-shorts and tiny tank tops are often the norm, whereas in predominantly straight locations members wear long baggy shorts and loose T-shirts or tank tops. It goes without saying that a member from one gym will clearly feel out of place at the other. Often, the mode of dress is affected by the weather and culture of the town: in Los Angeles or Miami, gyms—both gay and straight—are more skin-friendly than those in New York or San Francisco. This, however, is not always the case; in some cities the two very different environments are only one mile apart.

The popularity of the gay gym has resulted in a number of choices for gay men in dense urban areas, where we can now find different types of gay gyms. There are gay gyms that cater to the hip and young gay male; some are more popular with older males or bears; others are more mixed between gay and straight or men and women; some are lesbian only; some gay gyms are more social than others; some are notorious for the action one can find in the locker rooms; others are known for the opposite; some gay gyms are big-bodybuilder oriented; and others are more popular with the leaner athletic types.

MODERN GAY VS. STRAIGHT GYMS

The social dynamics are what make a gym gay. The biggest difference between gay and straight gyms is the type and amount of socialization that goes on.

Whether gay or straight, predominantly male-populated gyms are charged with testosterone. The difference is in how that testosterone is both directed and perceived. In a straight-gym environment, testosterone transforms the interactions into competitive and casual without a sexual nature. But in a gay gym, the testosterone takes its most naturally occurring course, and while competition between gay males is part of the equation, the sexual aspect of attraction toward the same sex assumes a stronger role. In straight men, masculinity is displayed as a sort of shield and protection; in gay men it is too, but it is also displayed and perceived as an invitation for sex. Basically, when sexuality enters the weight room, the potential for socialization increases dramatically. The same is true, of course, for predominantly heterosexual gyms that are coed, and when there is a healthy ratio of men to women, the amount and type of socialization turn the place into a meat market, just like most gay gyms.

In fact, the meat market environment of some straight gyms is one that many straight women prefer to avoid altogether. A big percentage of heterosexual females feel uncomfortable in a male-dominated gym environment. They feel exposed wearing just shorts and a T-shirt; they don't like to be seen when they're sweaty and clenching their faces as they push and pull the weights. Many opt for a women's-only gym, or, now that gay has become chic, many of these women prefer—you guessed it—a gay gym. For a similar reason many of them prefer to work out with a gay male trainer.

The level of intimacy in a gym can discourage socialization among straight men. Sometimes straight men will even avoid making eye contact with one another, lest someone think they're checking a man out. But when they are comfortable enough with their sexuality and their masculinity regardless of their sexual preference, the gym offers a fraternal bonding that is hard to find in other places. The higher the level of comfort, the more that competition turns into bonding and admiration. When this occurs, men feel more comfortable not just looking at one another, but also vocalizing their thoughts on one another's bodies. At this point it is not unusual for a man to express admiration for another, and even casually touch him (which, depending on the circumstances, can also express physical attraction). It is then not uncommon to find two straight men discussing each other's chest, arms, or legs—something that for the most part does not occur outside athletics and art, at least not between heterosexual men.

Something as simple as how gay men greet one another often differs depending on the environment they are in—more specifically, how gay or gay friendly that environment is. Greeting friends with a kiss or a hug is by and large a common greeting among gay men in urban centers, and this can present conflict in a very heterosexual environment where a handshake is the acceptable greeting. It goes without saying that it would be out of place for two men to greet each other with a kiss in a primarily male heterosexual gym. At a gay gym, or one that is mixed, the same scenario is accepted without hesitation. The level of comfort associated with touching and basic social interactions is one of the main reasons many gay men prefer a predominately gay gym.

For many straight men, the gym is only a place to work out, a tool they use, and it is completely separated from their social lives. For other straight men, socialization is part of the gym experience and they hang out with their buddies at the gym; but when it comes to dating or pursuing women, more often than not they have much better luck outside the gym. For gay men, on the other hand, the gym is a destination in itself. Of course, many gay men want to avoid socialization at the gym, but the gay gyms nevertheless present the option. The gay gyms are an extension of gay social life. The gym has become a meeting place for gay men; friends visit while working out, and gay couples will often meet each other at the gym after work or go to the gym together. The gym offers the opportunity to meet potential partners, whether for a long-term relationship or a single-serving one. For a straight man to pick up a casual female sex partner at the gym is rare—although as I am reminded by a female friend, "It doesn't stop them from trying." Whereas gay men, no surprise to anyone, do it all the time. In fact as we will examine in subsequent chapters, the possibility is at times what draws some gay men to the gym. Furthermore, as I will discuss in the locker room chapter (Chapter 12), the possibility of sex—right there and then—is sometimes also an option.

Gay and Straight

One of the most interesting dynamics of primarily gay or heavily gay-populated gyms of urban centers is the interaction between gay and straight men. Some gyms might be 90 percent gay, while others are split right in the middle. Regardless of the ratio, the places offer a social environment and opportunity for interaction that either group would most likely not put themselves in.

Gymnasiums, because of their association with the body at a most basic level, are very intimate places. It is exactly the intimate association with a gymnasium that can make some gay men very uncomfortable at a straight gym or straight men uncomfortable at a gay gym. However, if we cross the boundary, and this is happening quite a bit right now, the fear factor on both sides diminishes, and the alienation felt toward the other group diminishes as well. We start identifying as one and the same. In the socialization process, sexual preference becomes less relevant as we find other things in common. This is progress.

Another interesting dynamic has begun to evolve in the straight-gay social arena. At many mixed but heavily gay-populated gyms, it is often gay men who have the best-built bodies. This is cause for admiration (as well as envy) from other men—whether gay or straight. For the first time in modern history, straight men are starting to admire and even envy gay men on something so associated with masculinity—the male physique. This is, during our times, an unprecedented empowerment and equalizer for gay men and gay culture. The ripple effect of this cultural phenomenon is slowly participating in the deconstruction of divisive gay-versus-straight stereotypes and will no doubt have enormous weight on future generations.

The Future of the Gay Gym

Undoubtedly, the popularity of the gay gym will continue to increase among gay men in the near future. However, because of the assimilation of gay men into mainstream culture, it is likely that the social dynamics of gay gym culture will change and at some point the popularity of the gay-only gyms will begin to decrease (and this has already begun in New York and San Francisco). Of course, the result is largely subjective to geographic locations and the particular code of ethics for such locations. In sophisticated urban locations, where gay men continue to become part of the landscape, the need for gay-only gyms is not really as important as in a smaller city or town where gay and straight do not blend well.

When I moved into a new apartment in downtown San Francisco, I joined a gym across the street. On my first day there, I noticed that it was very mixed though leaning toward gay men. The same day, while I was working out, I ran into a straight male friend who gave me a quick account on the place:[9] "If you want mellow come in the late mornings and during the afternoon. If you want social, there are a lot more gay boys at night so the place tends to get more social and much more cruisy. And from what I've noticed, if you want to get some action, the steam room on Sunday afternoons . . ." and he starts to laugh and tells me, "You boys . . ." Of course, this was San Francisco, where many straight men and gay men are more and more comfortable sharing intimate social spaces, like gyms and even steam rooms. That the information I just referred to came from a straight male is a perfect example of how much gay and straight blend today. In direct contrast, I spent a few months in the Tampa Bay area of Florida, where I worked out at several suburban and predominantly straight gyms where gay and straight do not blend at all. It was painful for me to watch the uneasiness with which gay men—even the most "straight acting" ones—

carry themselves in less diverse and less sophisticated homophobic gym environments.

For gay men who live in suburbia, small cities and towns, and rural areas, the reality of gay gym culture is an option only when they travel to gay ghettos.

Regardless of what happens to gay-only gyms in the future, the influence that they have had in the building of a gay gym culture will continue to influence both gay and mainstream culture for a long time to come. The culture that was first established by the gay gyms now surpasses the geographical limits of the gay ghettos. The gay gyms will no doubt continue to set trends among gay men, and now that we live in the age of the Internet, gay mass media, and circuit parties, these trends will continue to stream out into the rest of gay culture.

Across socioeconomic levels, cultural, ethnic and racial lines, and age differences, gay men seem to have one thing in common: their attraction for muscle boys. This affinity for a well-muscled body is the one constant, which in turn, brings men of all ages, races, colors, and body shapes under one roof—the gym. The gym is one of those rare social establishments in gay culture today that actually houses such true diversity. Simply put, in urban America, being gay comes with a gym membership.

Chapter 6

Muscle Boys

Adam Boardman is a thirty-seven-year-old schoolteacher in San Francisco who has been working out for five years. When asked if he identifies with any of the other subcultures (bear, circuit, athlete, etc.) he states: "I'm just a regular guy, I don't fit neatly into any of these categories." When asked why he works out and goes to the gym, Adam says, "Probably the most obvious reason would be that as a gay man there's a certain amount of drive to look your best and to stay looking good as you get older."[1]

This chapter discusses guys like Adam, "regular guys" who go to the gym. In a paradoxical sense, the men in this chapter fit into a broader category, one that is not really about categories. In fact, the largest common denominators among the men in this large group are their age and their sexuality: they range in age from the late teens to the early forties, and in the online survey I conducted, most of them identify as "gay" or "bisexual" (89 and 9 percent, respectively) and a small percentage (2 percent) identify as "questioning" or "straight."

Men in this "no scene" category made up 46 percent of my survey respondents (see Figure 6.1). Of these, 39 percent claim no scene at all, and 7 percent elaborated on their answers giving us an interesting perspective on the gay identities of muscle boys. Of course, the term "regular guys" is a loose one, so I encouraged these guys to elaborate about their identities and lifestyles, and they gave me a long list of attributes that better describe who they are. The list proves that there really is no one category, but many, including: country western, military, bodybuilders, ravers, hippies, academics, radical-faeries, homebodies, Christians, musicians, jock-nerds, gay dads, urban hipsters, college frat scene, bi-guys, intellectuals, middle-class taxpayers, alternative tattoo dude, coupled-home-nesters, AA members, straight scene, black pride, urban-A-crowd, skinheads, porn stars, butch Latino homeboy,

Muscle Boys: Gay Gym Culture
Published by The Haworth Press, Taylor & Francis Group, 2008.
doi:10.1300/6034_06

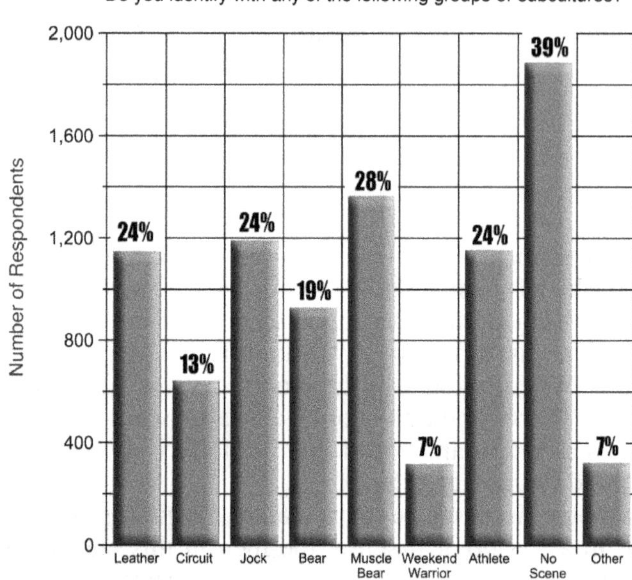

FIGURE 6.1. Association of gay gym culture to modern gay subcultures and stereotypes.

musical theater queen, etc. Although the list just about crushes stereotypical images about muscle boys, there are some important correlations that bring these men together under one roof—at the gym.

The involvement of these men in gym culture is heavily based on two factors: body image and socialization. This chapter will explore some of the basic topics within the realms of body image such as aesthetics, bodybuilding, and masculinity. I will also explore just how these images translate to determine socialization such as friendships, sexual encounters, dating, and long-term relationships. In addition, this chapter discusses how the variables within these two realms of self and social identity affect and influence the minds and bodies of gay and bisexual men today.

BODY IMAGE AND SOCIALIZATION

Brendan Eaton (a pseudonym), a magazine editor in Southern California, started working out when he was nineteen. Brendan is now twenty-five and working out has been a significant part of his adult life and gay experience. I met Brendan three years ago, when he was a student at the University of California, Berkeley, and noticed how, for him, the gym and working out are a very matter-of-fact part of his experience as a gay man. As he explains it:[2]

> It is as if everyone has realized that working out is important and your body is important and especially if you're worried about, you know, going out and looking good or meeting a partner or trying to be sexy, it is sort of accepted that what you need to do is go to the gym and work on your body. Because if you look around at the gay community, everyone—at least in this community here in Southern California—has made that such a focus. Almost everybody is going for that gym look, or that gym body, or trying to look muscular and attractive.

As we will discuss later, the circuit boy and the muscle bear maintain an image that is central to their social lives. But for the rest of the gay community, going to the gym and working out is fueled by a number of reasons, from the most simple to the very complex. What has become clear in my research and my own experience is that regardless of the diversity of these reasons, they will almost always fall into one of two categories:

1. *Body image:* aesthetics, sex appeal, bodybuilding, fashion/clothing, and masculinity—refers to the way we see and present ourselves physically.
2. *Socialization:* in gym culture refers to how self-image affects who we socialize with, and how this affects casual and serious relationships. Socialization determined by gym culture includes friendships, casual sexual encounters, dating, and life partnerships.

Although the body image and socialization of young gay males can be discussed as two isolated topics, when it comes to gay gym culture they are two issues that profoundly affect each other. Self-image determines socialization as much as socialization determines body and self-image, and in very few places is this more evident than in today's gay gym culture.

Building the Body Beautiful

What drives young gay men to go to the gym and sculpt their bodies? To answer the question, I interviewed and surveyed many gay men to get their insight, and the next few quotes mirror the answers of most:

> I want to look good in uniform.
>
> Twenty-seven-year-old in Pensacola, Florida

> To build confidence in myself. If I feel good about myself on the inside AND outside, then I gain confidence in the way I present myself in public . . . choosing to wear a tank shirt or tighter clothing. Men who are lean, muscular, in shape and take care of their bodies are just plain SEXY. The better I look, the less clothing I want to wear.
>
> Forty-year-old in Atlanta

> Appreciation of the male form, we're all jars of clay! Why not spice up my little neck of the woods for an undeterminable amount of time by getting chiseled at 6'1" and 185 lbs of pure, unadulterated testosterone and masculinity. That's why.
>
> Twenty-seven-year-old in Birmingham, Alabama

The major reasons young gay men go to the gym are to build muscle and to get leaner. Male beauty today in popular culture is largely defined by physical muscular symmetry. The symmetrical body characterized by a V-shape torso with broad shoulders and back, bulging pectorals, built arms, and a small and lean waist with long and muscular legs is today's definition of what makes a man physically beautiful. This body I am describing has also come to be known as the gym-built body, and clearly it is in pursuit of this physical shape that millions of young men—both gay and straight—hit the gym every day. Three men, who are in fact well built, illustrate this pursuit.

Complementing his all-American looks, Brendan already sports that gym body: his 5-foot, 10-inch frame is packed with 150 pounds of solid muscle, his body is chiseled, and he doesn't just have a six-pack, but an eight-pack. Yet for Brendan, his body is a work in progress:

> I think I would want more mass, because I'm lean. I don't want to look like a bodybuilder, but I want to look a little bit beefier, which means that I want my pecs to not just be chiseled but to actually come away from the body. I want bigger arms, bigger shoulders, and bigger legs . . . ultimately just more size.

Tom Madonna is a thirty-three-year-old leasing agent in San Francisco who has been working out for a year. Tom is not as interested in getting more muscular as he is in getting leaner. He tells me: "I was very happy with the results, because I changed my diet and started working out, and I lost twenty pounds of fat."[3] Although he feels more satisfied with his body than he was before, Tom also has some gym work left to do: "I just have that 2 percent body fat to drop, maybe another four or five pounds of fat."

When I ask Adam Boardman about his goals he tells me, "ideally I want bigger arms and chest and that's what I'm working toward."[4]

Just like Brendan, Tom, and Adam, 55 percent of the 5,576 men who took the survey reported using the gym to build muscle and 36 percent to get leaner or lose weight. The "gym body" is clearly what gay and bisexual men are striving to build at the gym (see Figure 6.2).

Body Image

Often when I read something about body image it is almost always accompanied by the word "obsession" it, as in "body image obsession." So often does body image get discussed only in terms of "obsession" that little is ever said about a healthy and normal body image, one that is not based on a pathological disorder but on normal wants and desires to be fitter or to look better. I am very familiar with eating disorders and body image pathologies such as muscle dysmorphia. These are serious and dangerous conditions. However, I also believe that the majority of people who work out and go to the gym on a regular basis do not come anywhere near pathology. There is a differ-

What are your reasons for working out or your involvement with the gym? (check all that apply)

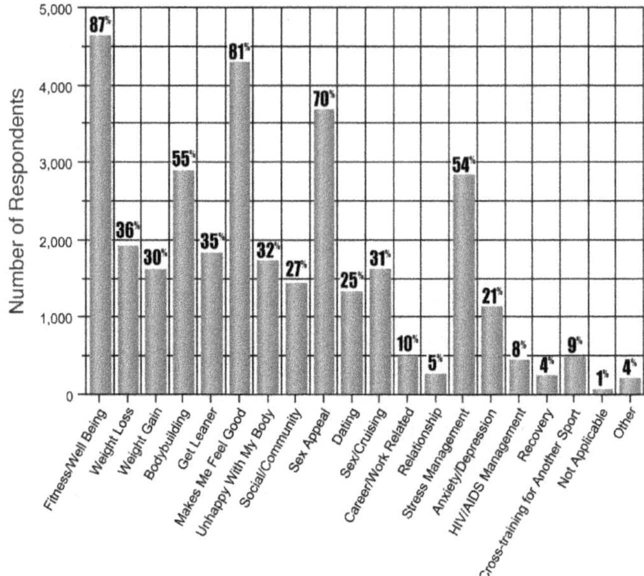

FIGURE 6.2. Breakdown of independent factors and goals that influence gay men to work out and/or get involved with the gym.

ence between being concerned with one's "body image" and wanting to look better versus being "obsessed" with it. One is normal and healthy; the other is not.

Sure, Brendan has specific goals as far as his body is concerned, but he is not losing sleep over it, as he tells me:[5]

> I'm happy with my body. I think there's always a part of me that wants to improve, and whenever I look at myself in the mirror or evaluate how I look, I always want more, I always want to be in better shape or to maybe have a little bit more size. So I don't think that ever goes away, but in general I'm happy with my body.

Many of the men I surveyed and interviewed shared with me their goals to build bigger pecs or arms or get that "six pack" or lose those ten pounds, but at the same time, the majority of them—a whopping 83 percent—also stated that they are generally satisfied with their

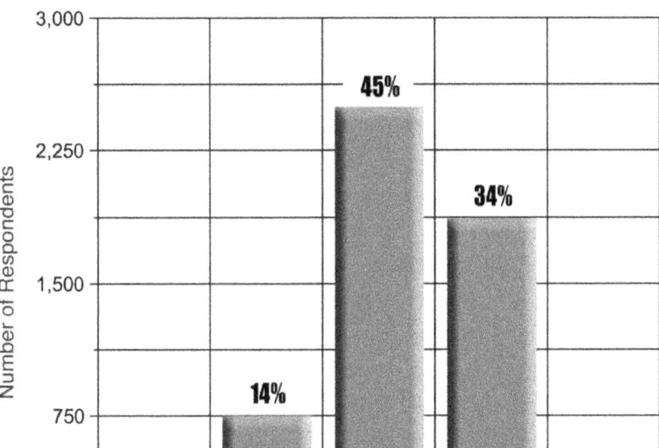

FIGURE 6.3. Levels of body image satisfaction within gay gym culture.

body. A minority of survey respondents, 17 percent, reported feeling "very unsatisfied," or "unsatisfied" (see Figure 6.3). The percentage of gay men satisfied with their body drops dramatically when we take into account those who do not exercise. A great deal of these unsatisfied men are the ones who checked the box "I do not work out" (4 percent of total survey respondents). What I found was a direct correlation between having a positive body image among those who exercise, and a less favorable one among those who do not.

Adam vacillates between feeling satisfied and not completely satisfied with his body, and is quick to point out that "I can definitely see things that I like to change about it, but it's not that important." What has changed for Adam, however, is how he feels about himself in relationship to his body:[6]

> It's made me more aware of the particulars of body image, instead of having a general self loathing. I like these things about my physical aspect. There are other things that I want to change, and this is how I can go about changing them. I know that if I break up things into small pieces, I can affect some change, and

> even the small amount of accomplishment gives me a sense of "Oh wow, my body looks better to me than it did nine months ago."

My personal training aesthetic is clearly defined by physical symmetry; however, it is also defined by a sense of wonder at the science behind human biodynamics and how beautiful and how perfect the human body is—regardless of its shape or age. An integral part of my personal training philosophy is based on teaching my clients the science behind exercise. A little bit of knowledge goes a long way in the development of a sense of respect for one's own body, which yields a healthier body image, not to mention a fitter and better looking body.

A lot of people hate their bodies, and this is the reason many of them join a gym. But I've learned that a few workouts, followed by even the slightest results, will begin to change a person's negative relationship to his or her own body. Something as simple as the muscular soreness that follows the first few workouts is a wake-up call, a reminder that hey, those are *my* muscles.

Working out regularly enhances body image in two ways: (1) the physical changes that create a better-looking body, and (2) the change in our relationship to our own bodies. As Adam tells me, aside from the physical changes that he feels make his body look better:[7]

> I really like the endorphin rush and the feeling that I get from going. I like going to the gym, but I really like afterward that sense of accomplishment. It's something I can control, I can get down there and I can do it and I can work out hard and feel like I've accomplished something. That's something that's been difficult for me all my life—to actually finish things that I start—so each step of going and working out and having a good workout and putting 100 percent into it is a minor victory for me.

COMPETING ON THE GAY MARKET AND SUCCESSFUL "MARKETING"

> I have to look at least as good as the competition!
>
> Forty-one-year-old in Norfolk, Virginia

The body beautiful plays a role in determining what is considered physically desirable. In a nutshell, building our bodies becomes an active effort to compete on the gay market and to successfully market ourselves.

Having a well-built body has become similar to having well-kept hair or dressing well. Basically, desirable and acceptable aesthetics for males have expanded to include muscular symmetry and definition. On the contrary, more and more, having a flabby and unkempt body is seen as stepping out with "bed head" and wrinkled clothes—neither aesthetically pleasing nor socially acceptable.

In fact, clothes very often are designed to improve the appearance of the body, to give it shape. A perfect example of this is the traditional man's suit, with its broad shoulders (often padded), giving the illusion of a V-shaped torso. This is one of the main reasons most people agree that men look good in suits and why it is the dress of choice for men to wear to business engagements and special social occasions. An interesting double standard is displayed by those people who criticize gym culture yet are immersed into fashion, which in itself is only a different type of body culture. Why anyone would think that it is appropriate and desirable for a man to wear a suit that will give his body the illusion of symmetry, but not desirable for that same man to actually build his muscles to have a more symmetrical body makes absolutely no sense.

A heavy preoccupation with aesthetics can no doubt lead to a level of narcissism that is not at all pretty, or healthy. Gym culture is one of the places where we can typically find young men who are so preoccupied with how they look as to not think of anything else—the definition of an excessive narcissist. But these men represent only a small percentage of gym culture and not the majority of gay men who go to the gym. Furthermore, narcissism is also found quite often outside and far and away from gym culture; it is not a modern gym culture phenomenon and has existed as far back as the myth from which the word takes its name. Freud explained that there are healthy levels of narcissism, and that it becomes pathological only when extreme and excessive, although most people attach only a negative correlation to the word. We need to differentiate between being concerned with aesthetics in a normal, acceptable, and healthy way, and that which is abnormal and harmful. To argue that aesthetics is the main reason young gay men are involved with the gym is not unreasoned, but to argue that the concern for aesthetics is pathological is—as Freud would agree—unfounded.

FITNESS AND HEALTH

Looking good is clearly a benefit that Brendan enjoys, but that is not all he gets from working out:[8]

> I work out because it makes me feel good about myself, not just because it improves my appearance. I've gotten used to the adrenaline rush. Taking time out of my day and working on my body and myself makes me feel good, and I like the way it makes me look. Also knowing that I'm doing something that's healthy for myself. I think it just feels really exhilarating after working out—you can't necessarily get that feeling doing anything else. I've seen progress, and once I started working out and got in a regular routine I probably was less involved in unhealthy activities. I stopped smoking.

Most of the men who participated in my survey seem to relate to Brendan's appetite for general fitness and health. In fact "fitness," and "well-being" turn out to be the frontrunner reasons why gay and bisexual men today are involved in the gym—a massive 87 percent (4,642) of survey respondents cited fitness and well-being as the driving forces behind their workouts (see Figure 6.2).

Generations "X" and "Y" grew up in eras when fitness and health were emphasized. Education about fitness and health begins as early as grade school and continues well into college. Apart from our system of education, fitness and health are also promoted by many other government agencies such as the Centers for Disease Control, the Surgeon General, the President's Council on Exercise, the American Medical Association, and the Federal Drug Administration, to name a few. There is in fact so much information out there promoting fitness and health that it is really difficult to open up a newspaper or turn on the television or the radio or go online without coming across a message reminding us to eat healthier and exercise.

Our parents and grandparents simply did not have the information that we have now; information was limited. The concept of exercise for its own sake seemed, and still seems, foreign to a lot of older people.

The importance of fitness and health, akin to ancient Greek times, has once again become part of a good education. Given what we know today about fitness and good health, there is absolutely no good argument as to why *not* to exercise. Like an education, fitness has understandably become something to strive for. Here we find another important correlation, and one that has been proven by researchers and scientists over and over: the higher the education level of any given group, the higher percentage of participants in fitness and athletic endeavors. As Figure 6.4 illustrates, the majority of survey respondents are college educated: 38 percent are college graduates and another 28 percent have graduate degrees. In this day and age, anyone who still believes the old "dumb jock" stereotype to be true, is really, really dumb.

In addition to fitness of the body, fitness of the mind is gaining momentum as a reason to work out. More and more, the field of psychology endorses exercise as a prevention and management strategy against depression and anxiety. Furthermore, many psychologists have gone as far as to question the efficacy of antidepressants when com-

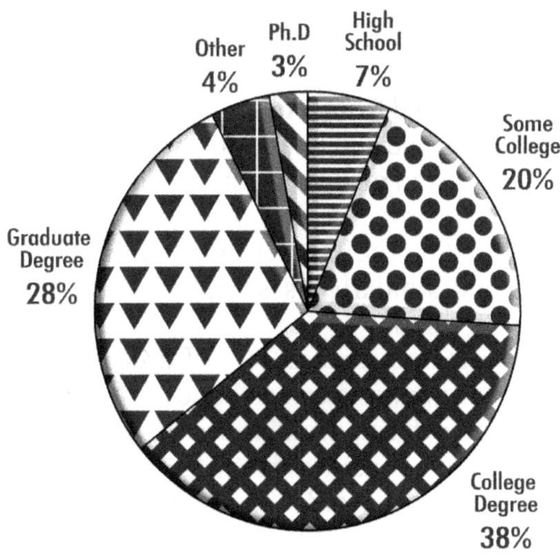

FIGURE 6.4. Gay gym culture education strata.

bined with an exercise program. Some speculate that improvement in patients' psyches is more a result of the exercise than antidepressants.

Fitness of the body is significantly connected to fitness of the mind, and while most young gay men do not pursue the gym out of concern for Zen, the connection is quickly made. Gay men initially pursue the gym out of a concern for aesthetics, but of the many other reasons that eventually become part of the fitness quest, the gym often becomes an outlet for managing stress, anxiety, and depression. Fifty-four percent of survey respondents reported using the gym and their workouts as a tool for "stress management," and 21 percent cited exercise in their quest to overcome and manage "anxiety and depression." Another smaller but sizeable contingent (5 percent or 278) reported using the gym to help them through one of life's toughest adversities: "relationship break-up." And, lastly, 10 percent (9.5 percent or 503) report the gym as another tool they use to enhance their jobs or careers (see Figure 6.2).

It has been well documented that gay males experience more anxiety and depression than their straight male counterparts. The creation of safe spaces for gay men to overcome anxiety and depression associated with coming out and self-esteem issues is an ongoing goal of the gay community. In the past two decades, the gym has become an important space for this. What happens is that the mind becomes centered, the body becomes buff, and at this point the outlet has turned into a lifestyle.

I have a dear friend and former client who is a Buddhist priest and a teacher of meditation; she and I have discussed at length the similarities between exercise and meditation and the positive effect that these can have on a person's psyche. She agrees with me that exercise is a different type of meditation, another type of mind-centering activity. This realization and similarity is something that many people are seemingly catching on to.

When I first started personal training I used to be concerned that my younger clients' emphasis on aesthetics was too great, and I tried unsuccessfully to preach health and fitness to the aesthetically driven. I realized that, like most advice given to the young, it was lightly taken. But I found that if I avoided the healthy body talk it was just a matter of time before clients would bring it up themselves. Instead of me telling them how they were going to be healthier, they were telling me how they felt healthier, how they were experiencing a sense of well-being they had not anticipated. Many were not just feeling better—they were feeling great. At this point, to pass on information and educate clients on human physiology and exercise science was a piece of cake; they were the ones probing me for information.

You've heard it over and over from those who exercise, but for the sake of statistics I had to ask. Eighty-one percent (4,301) of survey respondents reported using the gym and working out just because it "Makes me feel good" (see Figure 6.2).

BUILDING MASCULINITY

Masculinity is typically defined and understood to be characteristic male behavior, and unfortunately more often than not it is measured by half-baked methods, such as appearance, behavior, voice, and muscularity. Even before we are born, we are doctrined toward preconceived ideals of masculinity and femininity. Soon-to-be mothers shop for their unborn on the basis of their sex: blue if it's a boy, pink if it's a girl, thereby associating masculine or feminine traits (in this case colors) to an unborn child. Worldwide and across most cultures this practice happens in one way or another.

Ultimately, young boys come into a blue-colored, ball-playing, sports-minded environment even before they can tell the difference between male and female. Similarly, certain activities are associated with masculinity: weight training and bodybuilding. Weight training results in increased muscularity, which is typically seen as increased masculinity.

Throughout history, most heroes, warriors, champions, knights, and Samurais have been hypermasculine, well-muscled, strong, powerful men. In modern day, our idols and heroes have not changed much, either in appearance or in masculinity traits. In fact, traits of masculinity are now exaggerated in a way they have never been before (G.I. Joe, Arnold Schwarzenegger), and gay culture has not strayed behind (Tom of Finland, Colt). As I discuss in Chapter 4, like Tom's men and the men of Colt, today's hottest porn starts and other gay male objects of desire are extremely built and muscular men.

Interestingly enough, even though it was not a question I asked on my initial surveys or interviews, masculinity was often cited as an answer in relationship to how working out influenced self-image. "I feel more masculine," was often cited with a generalized assumption that feeling more masculine was a benefit and/or improvement. In fact, masculinity kept coming up over and over in survey after survey and interview after interview when the topic of self-image was discussed, and more specifically when I asked young men the question: "How has participation in the gym affected your self-image?"

During my research, the assumption that increased masculinity was a good thing was so pervasive that on several occasions when I asked the interviewee to elaborate on his answers, he would often look at me with a puzzled expression of "I have to explain it to you?" Masculinity in relationship with gym involvement was such an influencing topic that before conducting my survey online I added the following questions:

1. How important is it for you to (behave and appear) masculine?
2. How important is it that the men you're attracted to appear and behave masculine?

Answers to both questions reveal that, for gay and bisexual men today, masculinity is, for the most part, a nonnegotiable demand whether from potential partners or from ourselves. As Figure 6.5 illustrates, when answering the first question "How important is it for you to (behave and appear) masculine?" the majority of respondents (68 percent) list masculinity to range from "important" (28 percent), to "very important (24 percent), and "extremely important (16 percent). And when it came to the second question, "How important is it that the men you're attracted to appear and behave masculine?" masculine behavior and appearance assumes an even higher premium: 75 percent of the respondents said that it is "important" (28 percent), "very important" (29 percent), and "extremely important" (18 percent).

Having learned from my earlier survey that masculinity as a topic would invite large interest, I also posed the question "In your mind what defines masculinity?" allowing respondents to "check all that apply" from a long list of common masculine-associated traits (see Figure 6.6).

My findings illustrate how we measure masculinity by "half-baked" measures. "Behavior" clearly leads how masculinity is defined, yet "behavior" is another one of those million-dollar words that truly has not one but countless definitions. The truth is, as a twenty-

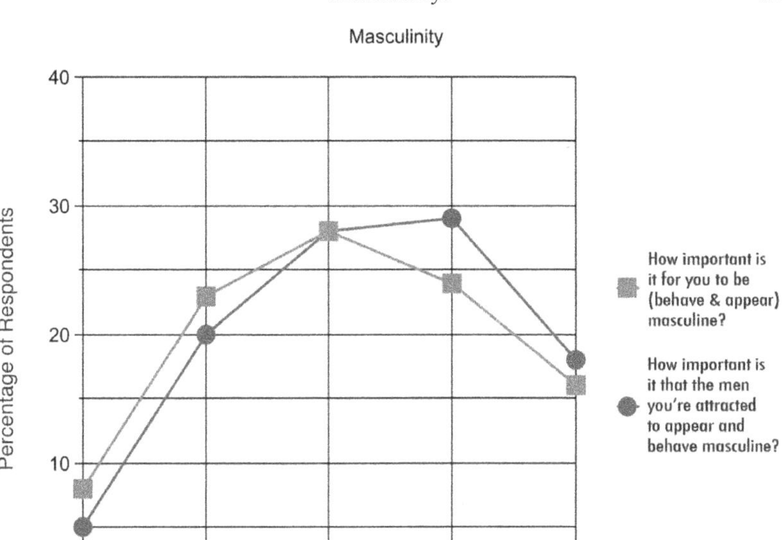

FIGURE 6.5. Masculinity: levels of importance given to masculine appearance and behaviors in modern gay gym culture.

eight-year-old business owner in Kansas wrote about masculinity when taking my survey:

> It's a cliché expression that doesn't mean anything any more. What is masculine to one means nothing to another. It's so arbitrary. I only know what I am attracted to.

Yet, it is also true that half-baked or not, many of these measures and characteristics not only have powerful influence but will continue to define masculinity. Furthermore, how masculinity is perceived and defined will also continue to change and evolve with time, culture, and fashion. When I was a kid, for example, using hair gel was not considered masculine, but today (and only some twenty years later) it is hard to find a modern man who leaves the house without gel, mousse, paste, pomade, or whatever type of gunk he puts in his hair.

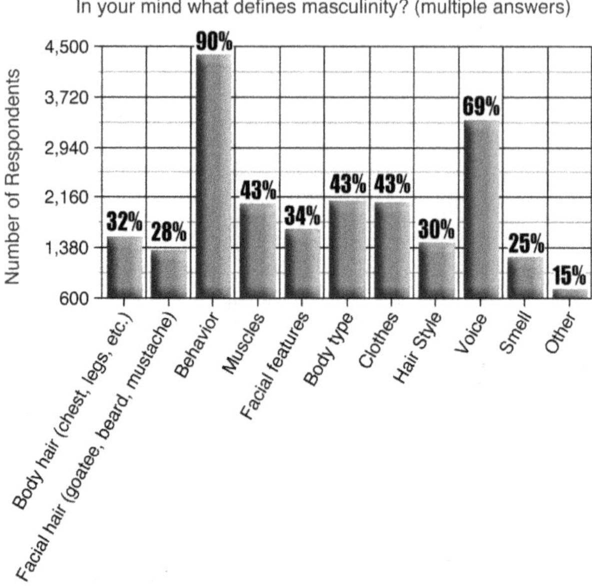

FIGURE 6.6. Masculinity: defining traits in modern gay gym culture.

The masculinity associated with a muscular V-shaped torso is also—it turns out—a serious driving force for young gay men hitting the gym. Messages idealizing masculinity in gay men are everywhere, from the poetry of Homer to the personal ads on Gay.com. This of course can be problematic, because for some gay men masculinity does not come so naturally. Historically, this is nothing new: masculinity has been a desirable trait for young males since history has been documented. What is novel here is the concept of the masculine gay male.

Many gay young men refer to athletic masculinity as a "look" or an "appeal" that they can connect to and identify with by going to the gym and working out; as Brendan Eaton points out: [9]

> There are a lot of men, I think, who have this masculine appeal because they work out, they're athletic. I think that going to the gym has helped me see that I too can participate in a sport; I can body build and have that same sort of look and express my mas-

> culinity that way, instead of some of the more traditional ways like playing football.

The message is clear in modern gay culture: the most desirable males are muscular and masculine. Not a problem: muscular can be built, and masculine can be learned. Muscularity is defined by a set of muscles that have been built into symmetrical shapes. Masculinity is a set of skills, which is easier to learn for some men than others; nevertheless it is still a learned behavior. Today, the gym has, of course, become another tool into the acquisition of these sets of muscles and set of skills.

The connection between the gym and athletics and masculinity opens up the doors for young men like Brendan to get in touch with their masculine side: [10]

> I think there's an understanding that being masculine has always been equated a lot with how good you're at sports, and your mannerisms and stereotypes about being gay. I wasn't really athletic, and I didn't have a real athletic body—not that I'm extremely feminine—I'm sort of in the middle. So going to the gym and getting that more athletic look and actually doing something physical and doing hard work at the gym . . . it touches on a masculine side of you. You feel that you're doing things that masculine men have been doing for a long time. It is a way of participating in that.

The desire to appear the alpha male is so powerful that simply walking into the gym causes some men to immediately adjust their body language. Both masculinity and muscularity are displayed by an exaggerated military torso position characterized by sticking out the chest, pulling the shoulders back, and holding the arms a few inches away from the sides of the body. This position, of course, simulates those men who have very muscular torsos. This is an interesting display of body language, especially when it is displayed by men who lack the muscle mass.

Furthermore, the voice deepens and words like "dude" and "bro" come out the mouths of men who typically refer to their friends as "girl." Again, it should be made clear that while this body-language behavior takes place among gay men, it happens just as much if not more with straight men. But the transformation from a *hey-girl* personality to a *yo-dude* one never fails to amaze me, especially when it happens during the sixty seconds that it takes to get out of the car and walk into the gym.

Many gay men adjust their level of displayed masculinity according to their environment. I have watched the same man consistently behave differently at two different gyms in the same week. This is a survival mechanism that invariably protects some gay men from ridicule or even physical attacks when engaged in a hypermasculine and sometimes homophobic environment. On many levels, the hypermasculine body language is a display of gym fear. It displays just how uncomfortable some men feel at what they perceive as an evaluation of their masculinity.

When it comes to masculinity and internalized homophobia, the gym clearly keeps the two connected, yet the gym can play two very different roles. On the one hand, it can help men overcome internalized homophobia as they become more comfortable with themselves and their own level of masculinity and that of others. For most men, a few workouts are more than enough to realize that this *hypermasculine* perceived activity of lifting weights is something they can do regardless of how masculine they might be—that there is really nothing to it. On the other hand, the high level of idealized masculinity can make some men feel completely alien to the environment, resulting in a lot of *straight-acting* behavior and a constant sense of not fitting in, both of which can deepen their own insecurities and intensify their feelings of internalized homophobia.

Still, gyms are generally friendlier toward gays than in the past; as Brendan points out:[11]

> Once you see that a lot of gay men are doing it and going, you don't have to feel self-conscious in the gym. You go to any gym and a large part of it is gay; even at a straight gym there are always gay people working out. There's just something about being physical and doing physical activity and working hard that can make you feel you've done something more masculine.

Other gay men feel that masculinity and the gym have very little to do with each other. Adam feels that:[12]

> My ideas of masculinity don't have anything to do with the physical. I think there are stereotypes and icons of masculin-

ity—sort of big, super, buff, muscle guys, but my own feeling of what is sexy and masculine has much more to do with something that is coming from the inside of that person, a level of self-confidence or the way the person carries himself. To me really masculine guys have not necessarily been muscle-bound-he-men.

Adam is right, because in many ways masculinity really is an indescribable quality.

Finally, there is an important factor in the presentation and acceptance of masculinity in modern times that only complicates how we both perceive it and display it: we now live in a feminist-positive world that, at times, is overly sensitive to and chastises all that is masculine. Why is it that young gay men are encouraged to get in touch with their feminine side (which is not always part of our nature), but if we try to get in touch with our masculine side (which for the most part is) we get crucified for it?

BUILDING COMMUNITY

> I use the gym quite intentionally to socialize and to develop a circle of loose-knit friends. My close friends, college friends, are almost to a letter not athletic or into the bar scene much at all. So I have used the gym to find guys who share some of those interests, especially when I relocated from Minnesota to Utah. The gym helps me connect to the gay community, and a part of the community that I enjoy, more easily than doing it online or at the bar. (Forty-one-year-old in Utah)

When I asked Brendan Eaton if the gym played a part in his social life, he is quick to answer: "Yes, very much so. I think it's a place to be social, I've met a lot of friends there. I have dated men from the gym."[13] Like Brendan, 27 percent (or 1,445) of the men who took my survey reported using the gym as a social outlet or place for community (see Figure 6.2).

> I work out for physiological and psychological benefits, but I choose a (predominantly) gay gym for social/community reasons. I do go to circuit events and clubs occasionally, but the

> gym is the center of my social life. Most of my friends are there. It is where social plans are made and networks are strengthened. I like going when the gym is most crowded because I like visiting with people. I usually stay about one and a half hours but only really work out about 45 to 60 minutes. (A thirty-nine-year-old in Atlanta)

Concerns with self-image such as aesthetics and masculinity are important to young men because it affects and to a great extent largely determines their socialization. Although the gym itself often becomes a social outlet, participation in the gym will still determine social ties outside the gym—even when any type of social interaction is completely absent. For purposes of this chapter, I refer to socialization as those social interactions that occur either in the gym or outside it but are in one way or another connected by body image or awareness whether directly or indirectly.

As a personal trainer I will be the first to tell you that so much socialization goes on at the gym that it gets in the way of the workouts. Some men who socialize heavily will spend two or three hours at the gym to complete a workout that could be accomplished in forty-five minutes. This is the reason many gay men prefer to go to a gym with little or no socialization. I have a friend who after about two years at the same gym would switch membership to a new gym where he did not really know that many people, for the simple fact that he would spend so much time chatting with people.

Yet, the fact that we are there to work out is what makes the gym an appealing social outlet. When we walk into a bar, socializing is expected, and this expectation is enough to make a lot of people nervous and even uncomfortable. At the gym however, the focus of the activity is working out, yet we have the option to socialize while we are there. The option presents an ideal setting for many young gay men who feel uncomfortable in other social settings.

When you ask most people why they started going to the gym, the answer often involves a personal relationship: "I went with a friend" or "I was dating this guy who worked out and I went with him." At other times, the reason is very similar to the reasons we do a lot of things: because everyone else is doing it.

As with any other activity, once an interest in the lifestyle built around working out has been identified, we begin to look for and associate with those who share the same interests; in this sense gym culture is not much different from a book club or a bowling club. Because we are social animals, forming friendships and groups around similar interests is second nature to most of us. Of course this happens with any type of interest, but when it comes to gym culture it is easily identifiable because the gym-built body is often obvious. There is no obvious way to know that some guy who walks into a pub or a party is into bowling or the opera, but if he is gym built, the shape of the body is often an obvious description of at least some of his interests. Muscle boys are easily identifiable; the identification will give rise to a number of different feelings in others, feelings that range anywhere from camaraderie to desire to envy.

For Brendan, the gym has basically always been a part of his adult life. For Tom and Adam however, joining the gym is something that they struggled with because they did not identify with gym culture. Prior to the past year in which he has made the gym a part of his life, Tom Madonna tells me that: [14]

> I've never been the type to be into gym culture, and I really looked down on it. And a lot of the reasons I looked down on it, and probably why a lot of gay men do, is because they don't fit in, they don't have the body. So I was anti-gym. But now I'm a lot more open minded and I'm a lot more educated about the reasons people go to the gym.

Tom's prior sentiment toward the gym is something that Adam used to also mirror:[15]

> For years, there was no way I was going to have anything to do with the gym. When I started, I would ask myself, "Why am I going to go to the gym, seeing these people I don't want to see?" I was covering up for my own fear about things that I didn't understand or was relating to on a level of high school athletics. But once I was in a situation where I was going on a regular basis, it was like, "Oh, it's just a bunch of guys, it's not that big of a deal."

Adam feels different about "these people" these days; in fact, not only does he like them, he feels that interacting with them even on a very casual basis has changed his outlook on his sense of community and certain social situations:

> Working out and seeing other guys gives a sense that there are a lot of gay men who have gone through experiences similar to what I've gone through. I'll go somewhere and there'll be this shirtless muscle boy who'll be like, "Oh hey, how are you?" and my friends are like, "Who the hell was that?" It has made me more comfortable because I'll run into people I have a tenuous acquaintanceship with. It has opened me up to a certain amount.

Friendships between men who work out are common; there is a sense of camaraderie that is built by the gym regardless of how much one socializes there. Tom Madonna tells me that after only a few months at his gym, he already recognized at least half of the other gym members. This familiarity opens up the doors for further socialization. Brendan feels that the camaraderie is:[16]

> . . . something specific with the gym, is being able to develop relationships with men. One thing that it has done, is that it has created an environment in which I can interact with heterosexual men and feel comfortable.

SEX, DATING, AND RELATIONSHIPS

Some casual friendships form and others flourish at the gym, but when it comes to more intimate relationships, such as those of a sexual or romantic nature, the gym and gym culture have a greater impact on the men we choose to date, have sex with, and partner up for long-term relationships.

Seventy percent (3,695) of the men who answered my survey reported using the gym to enhance or build sex appeal. In most humans, the building of sex appeal has only one goal in mind: to enhance social and sexual situations, period. More specifically, 25 percent (1,329) of respondents cited using the gym in association with "Dating," and 31 percent (1,622) of them cited "Sex and Cruising," as their reasons for gym involvement (see Figure 6.2).

For Brendan:[17]

> Now that I've gone to the gym and I've worked on my body, if I was to date somebody who didn't put any effort into his body and didn't have enough of what I consider appealing I would

> probably be less interested in him. Before, I might not have noticed it so much because there wasn't so much contact with my own personal goals with my body.

The best and most blunt examples of this kind of selection process can be easily observed by logging on to any of the popular gay dating or sex hook-up Web sites popular today. Nowhere is the message that "bigger is better" laid out more directly than online. Surf through the personal ads on PlanetOut.com or Gay.com or on a sex hookup Web site like m4m4sex.com or manhunt.net and 90 percent of the personal ads are mostly about chest size, waist size, thigh size, bicep size, penis size—it's all about size, size, size. So much importance is placed on the built muscle body that pecs, triceps, and abs are becoming the crucial statistics young gay men are using to describe and define themselves.

Of course, prejudice isn't only about size. Some online profiles and magazine or newspaper personals include the phrase "no fats or fems." This is an embarrassing display of the internalized homophobia and the lack of sensitivity and political correctness that the male gay community displays in its most hypocritical moments. Two things, however, need to be made clear: (1) the offensive phrase is not necessarily the product of gym culture (as it is often blamed), and, (2) it was prevalent before gym culture. In fact, the phrase is quite often found in the profiles of gay men who have never set foot in a gym—and never will.

What is problematic with the "bigger is better" mentality is that even if we do not share the philosophy, it is hard to escape it. Before I started working on this book, I was doing triathlons and training a total of twelve to fifteen hours a week on endurance sports plus my four or five weekly weight-training workouts. Once I started the book, I discontinued the endurance training and kept only the gym workouts. In the process, I bulked up from 175 pounds to 200, and basically went from having the lean body of a triathlete to the bulkier and buffer body of a bodybuilder. The change was noticed by friends and acquaintances, most of whom complimented me on the bigger body. Even though on an intellectual level I do not subscribe to the "bigger is better" mentality, every time someone tells me that I look better being bigger I am tempted to believe it a little bit more.

We like to tell ourselves that size doesn't matter because it is the politically correct thing to say. Reality is much different, and those who really believe that size doesn't matter are either ignoring reality or just not paying attention. The following has become almost a proverb in gay culture, "there are two types of gay men: size queens and liars."

This is a touchy subject, because of course many people feel excluded, yet it is what is happening. As unfortunate as it is, I am quite sure that it is not going to change dramatically any time soon. There is something to be said for physical attraction: it is what brings people together in the first place. As Brendan also points out:[18]

> I think it would be nice to be interested in someone because they're intelligent, they're interesting, they're funny, but it's just that those things aren't always the most important, at least in the beginning.

The division that body image creates in gay culture is something that men who participate in it are clearly aware of and something that a lot of us are more sensitive to. Meanwhile, 44 and 47 percent of the men I surveyed stated that their involvement in the gym has changed the expectations of the men they date and have sex with, respectively; the majority of them, 76 percent, stated that it does not affect their friendships (see Figure 6.7).

While Tom says he believes in having a well-rounded group of friends, he also recognizes that:[19]

> Once you start feeling better about yourself, you do feel a little elitist, you do get a little judgmental. You think well, "I'm taking the time out to do this, this is not easy, sometimes it's not fun. I'm in pain the next day because of working out. So therefore, why can't you do it?"

When I ask Tom how he might feel judgmental he tells me that for example, earlier that day:

> I was walking behind this guy who probably could be really good looking. He's walking his cute little dog, wearing a cool T-shirt, he totally thought the outfit through—accessories, his hair looked good. But he had this fat under the chin, and from behind you can see the love handles, and I looked at him and I thought, "You know, it's funny, it's really easy to put on an out-

fit, it's really easy to put a look together and get the right accessories, but he looked really unhealthy to me; he didn't look like someone I would want to be intimate with, or see naked. Not that I wouldn't be friends with him . . ."

The reality is that like Tom, many of us vacillate between paying attention to the barriers created by body image, and aiming for inclusiveness, while actively putting up bricks for the wall. Is Tom being prejudiced? Yes, but he also has a really interesting point: while one can't help one's height or skin color, one can keep oneself fit. There are shades of gray in prejudice. In modern times, it is an acceptable given that for successful relationships similar levels of education and income are desirable from our partners, why then shouldn't it be reasonable to have expectations of a persons' body, given the fact it is actually the vessel of intimacy and sex?

Of course, relationships are a difficult process, and finding common ground is crucial in the success of a relationship. Working out

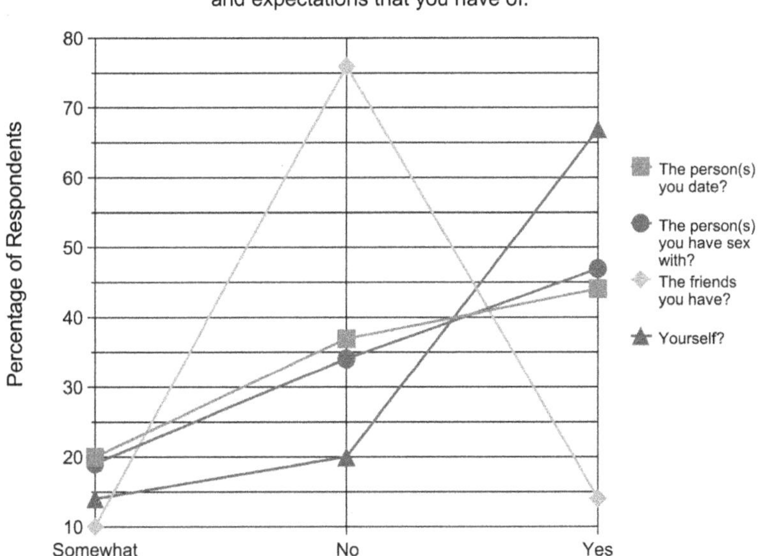

FIGURE 6.7. How gay gym culture alters and influences standards and expectations in relationship to modern gay self-image and interpersonal relationships.

and having successful results demand a healthy lifestyle that expands beyond the bench press and the Stairmaster. Staying in shape requires thoughtful shopping and cooking, getting enough sleep and rest, and working out often enough to see results. These steps take up a substantial amount of a working man's free time. Men who take training seriously have taken the effort to build their lifestyles around working out, and this can become problematic when they're dating someone who has a very different lifestyle and different set of priorities. Something as simple as cooking together and sharing a meal can become an issue if one partner is interested in healthy eating and the other wants fat-laden gourmet, or if one partner spends two hours at the gym and the other one spends two hours at the local bar for happy hour.

Of course, there are many gay men who work out *only between* boyfriends. Sometimes, they are the ones who get most frustrated with gym culture because the gym becomes something they feel they should do, and not something they want to do. In addition, they never stick to the gym long enough to see lasting results. Some men work out more often or work out only when they have a boyfriend or partner who does. For these men, working out becomes an integral aspect of having a relationship; it is how they spend quality time together

However, most young men involved with the gym work out regardless of whether they are single or partnered. As my findings demonstrate, many are interested in dating only men who also work out. Interestingly enough, a small proportion of men in the San Francisco survey I conducted stated that gym involvement could influence expectations of those they have sex with but not necessarily those they date, as if sex and dating were mutually exclusive.

No Pain, No Gain

Often when we begin working out seriously, we understand the amount of work and energy and sometimes pain that is required to build a muscular body. There is a certain amount of truth to the old bodybuilding slogan, "No pain, no gain." Weight training that yields results requires consistent time, sweat, and pushing our limits. It is hard physical work. (Of course, difference should be made between pain associated with soreness, which is a desired outcome, and pain associated with injury, which is not.) A few tough workouts are enough to begin to appreciate how hard and how much work it has taken those in better shape to get there.

On an intellectual level, we can compare the building of a beautiful body to that of getting an education. Education is something that takes time, energy, and dedication. One is not simply granted a college degree—one has to earn it. Similarly, most of us do not have naturally sculpted muscular bodies—we have to build them.

GETTING PUMPED UP

One of the best indications of how much body image is tied to a young man's self-image and his socialization is to watch his progression once he joins the gym. I've had clients who after only two or three workouts begin to see results. There is an explanation for this: during a workout, the muscles being worked out use a lot more blood than normal, so blood goes from the internal organs to the muscles, literally "pumping" them up. This "pumped up" effect will give an impression that the muscles are larger for the next couple of hours until the blood goes back to its normal function. The pumped-up look is a temporary illusion, but its influence on the mind is not. In addition, on the hormonal level, the body will start producing more testosterone and endorphins; the increased hormones will result in increased energy, libido, and feelings of well-being—all of which quickly translate into increased self-confidence.

The "pumped up" effect is so effective that almost immediately it will begin to change a young man's relationship to his body and his relationship to gym culture. In my experience, it is typically a change for the better. Someone who is not proud of his body and prefers to cover it up as much as possible during the first few workouts at the gym—by wearing long sleeves and sweats—will begin buying and wearing tank tops and shorts. In other cases, someone who might have been intimidated by others at the gym, or felt excluded from those who work out, begins to socialize and identify with them. Eventually, we figure out that the pumped-up illusion is only temporary, but if we stick with the workouts, by this point the muscles have quantifiably grown and our hormonal levels of testosterone are relatively higher on a constant basis. By then, the illusion is no longer "snake oil" and our minds and bodies are—literally—pumped up.

The pumped-up muscles and pumped-up hormones have such a powerful effect on the mind and the body, that, in my opinion, it creates a strong desire to exercise. Unlike an external effect (such as a "hot" picture on a magazine), here the effect is internal; it is happening within ourselves. The positive feelings associated with the effects will have a profound and lasting effect much more powerful on a physical and psychological level than most external influences such as cash, cars, clothes, or boys.

The gym offers gay men a place of community, a healthier alternative to bars and nightclubs, while at the same time giving them a piece of the gay culture social pie. But getting "pumped up" is the realization of all the influencing factors I discussed in this chapter—it is sexuality; aesthetics, confidence, masculinity, and desirability come together in one.

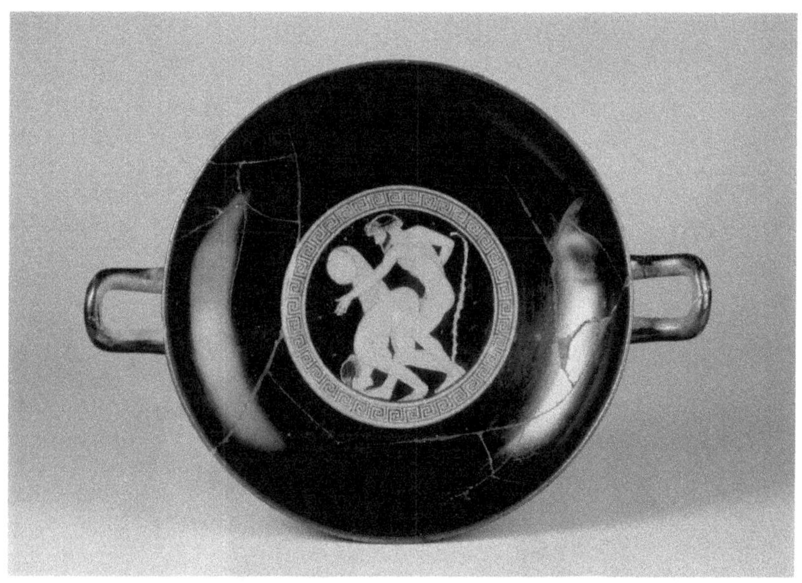

PLATE 2.1. Red-figure kylix decorated with a homoerotic scene by Briseis Painter (Fifth Century BC), Ashmolean Museum, University of Oxford, UK/The Bridgeman Art Library.

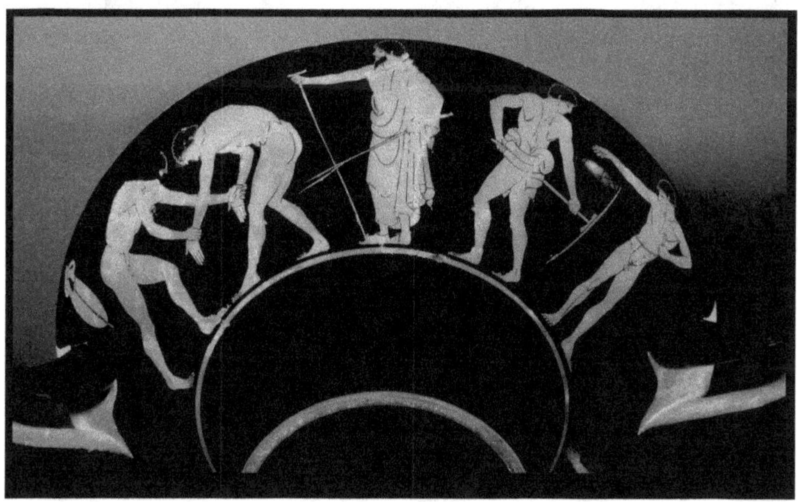

PLATE 2.2. Attic red-figure kylix depicting athletes training (Fifth Century BC), Ashmolean Museum, University of Oxford, UK/The Bridgeman Art Library.

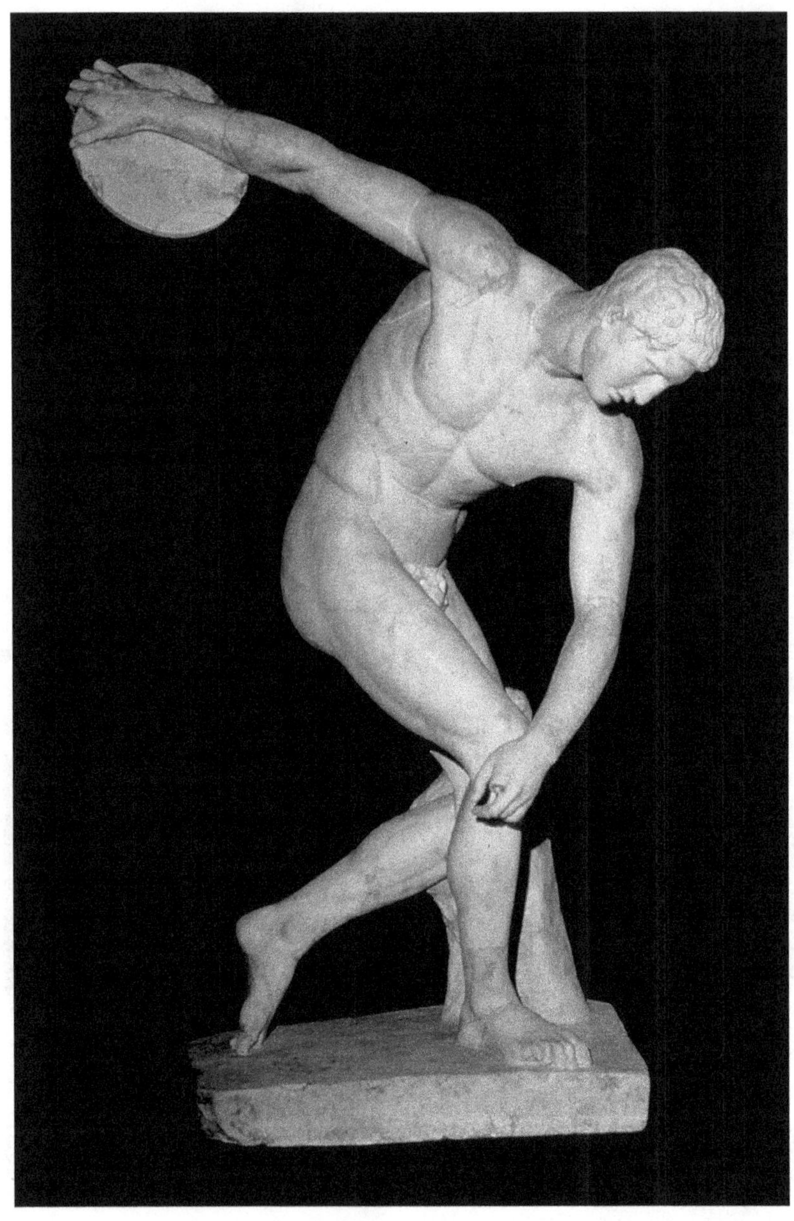

PLATE 2.3. Discobolus (marble) by Myron (fl.c.450 BC) (after), Location Unknown/Ancient Art and Architecture Collection Ltd./The Bridgeman Art Library.

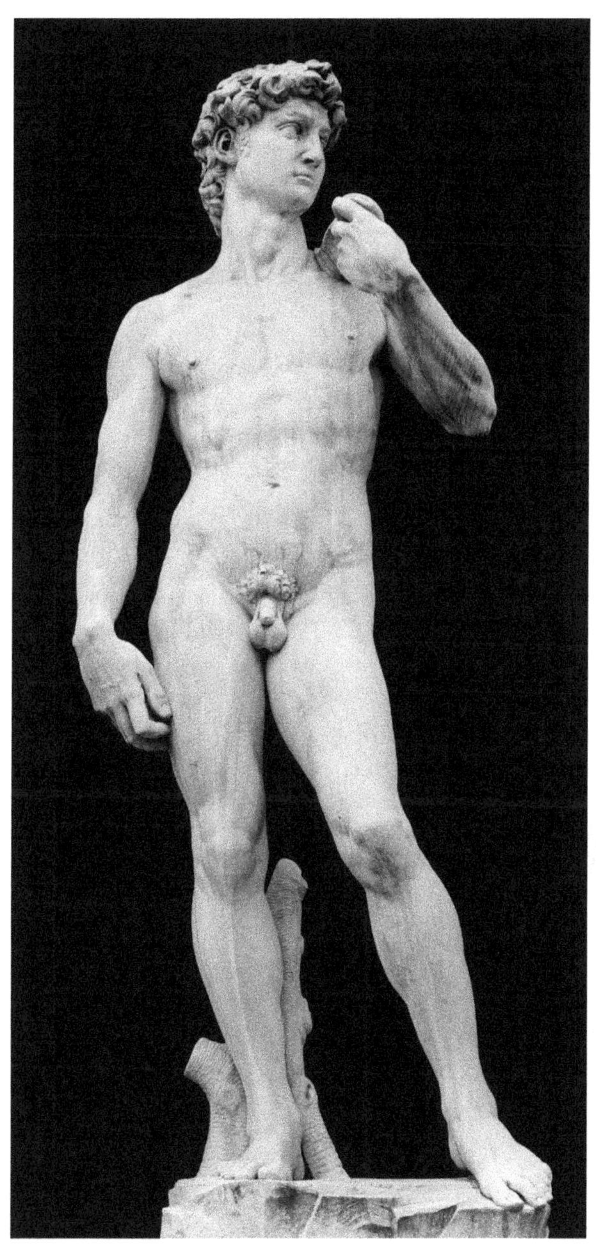

PLATE 3.1. Statue of David, Michelangelo. © iStockPhoto.com.

LOUIS CYR,
POLICE GAZETTE CHAMPION HEAVY LIFTER
OF THE WORLD.

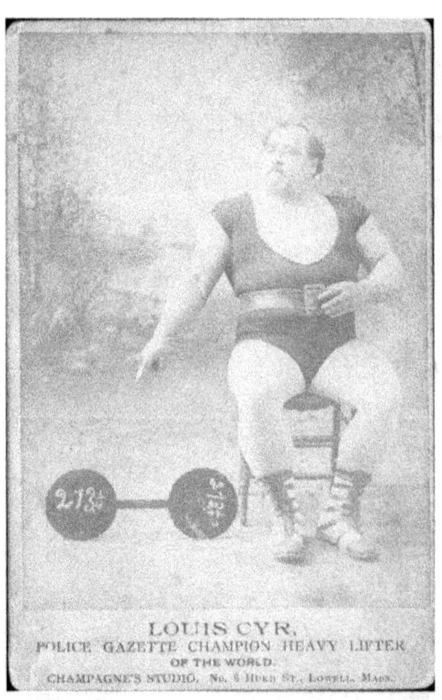

PLATE 3.2. Louis Cyr, famous nineteenth century strongman, Cabinet card (1900). Courtesy of The Magazine Archives, San Francisco.

SANDOW
Sandow.
182 REGENT ST. W.

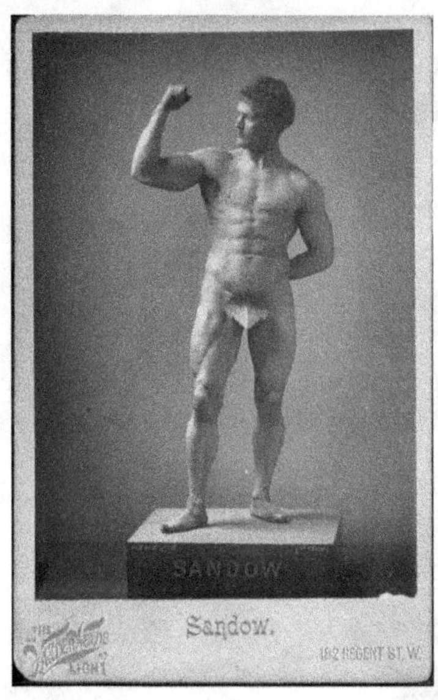

PLATE 3.3. Eugen Sandow, father of bodybuilding, by Van der Weyde, Cabinet card (1894). Courtesy of The Magazine Archives, San Francisco.

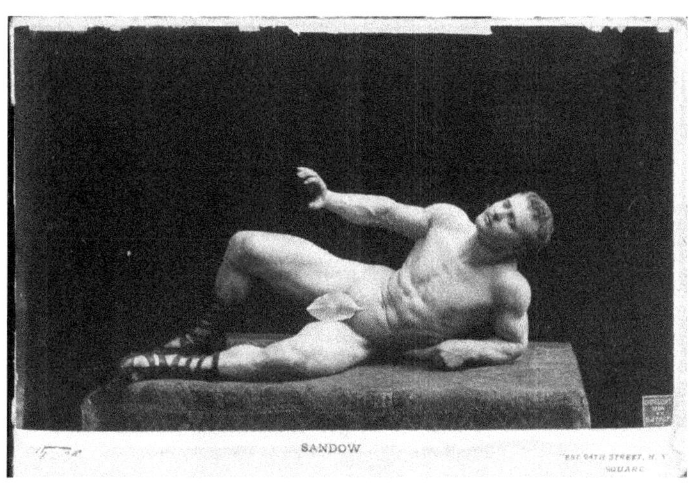

PLATE 3.4. Eugen Sandow, by Falk, Cabinet card (1894). Courtesy of The Magazine Archives, San Francisco.

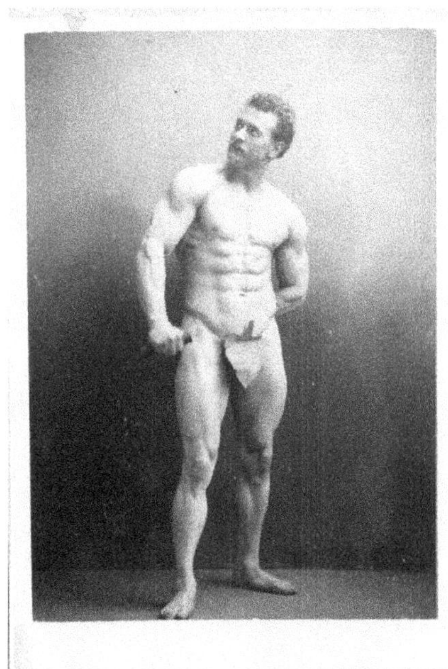

PLATE 3.5. Eugen Sandow, by W. Brooks, Cabinet card (1915). Courtesy of The Magazine Archives, San Francisco.

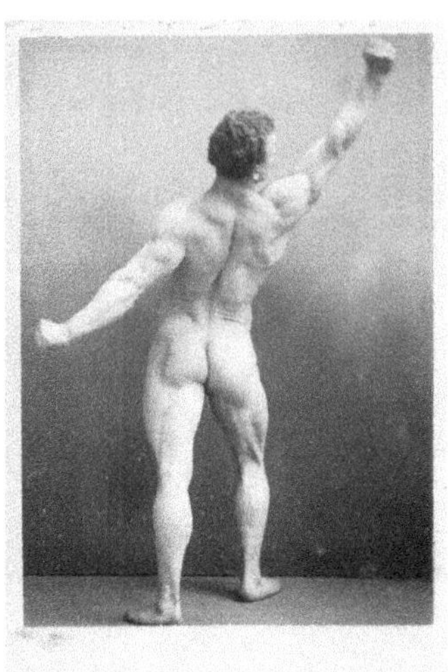

PLATE 3.6. Eugen Sandow, by W. Brooks, Cabinet card (1915). Courtesy of The Magazine Archives, San Francisco.

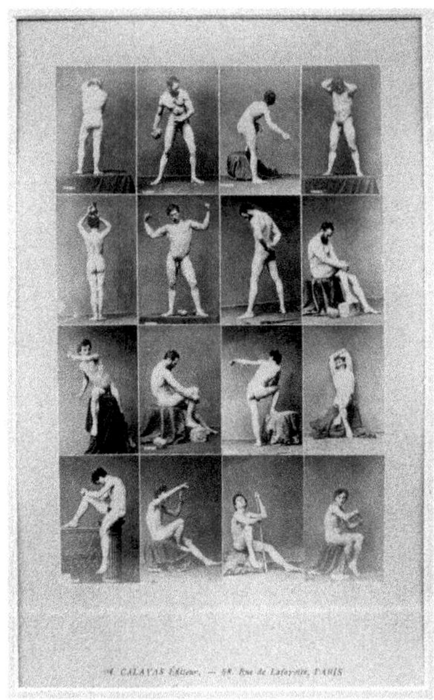

PLATE 4.1. A. Calavas, French albumen print page of photographic figure studies from a folio (1865). Courtesy of The Magazine Archives, San Francisco.

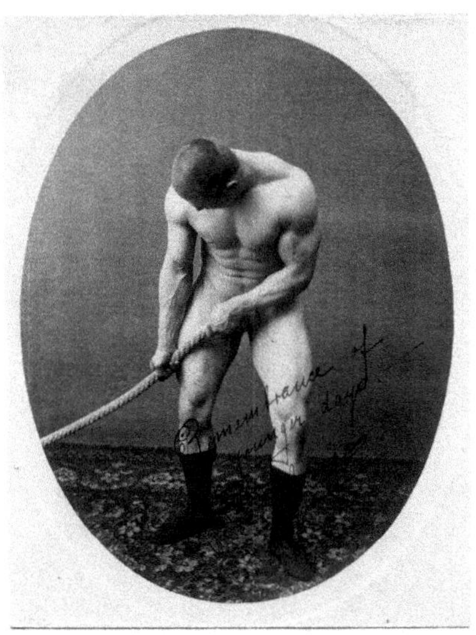

PLATE 4.2. George Hackenschmidt, famous wrestler and bodybuilder; photographer unidentified (1900). Courtesy of The Magazine Archives, San Francisco.

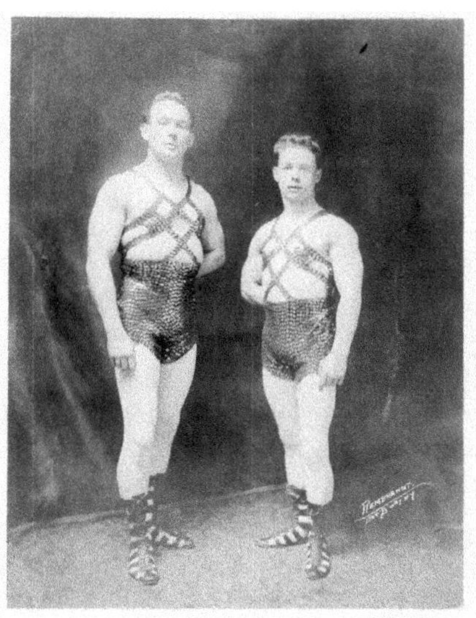

PLATE 4.3. Roland Brothers, probably a vaudeville act, by Rembrandt Studio, NYC (1910). Courtesy of The Magazine Archives, San Francisco.

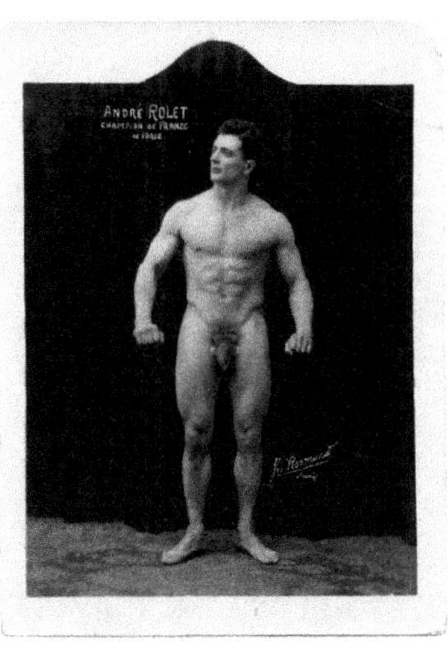

PLATE 4.4. Andre Rolet, French bodybuilder (photo is marked "Jos Rosmand, Paris" on front but stamped "Photo Studio Armand Leflohic, Paris" on back) (1930). Courtesy of The Magazine Archives, San Francisco.

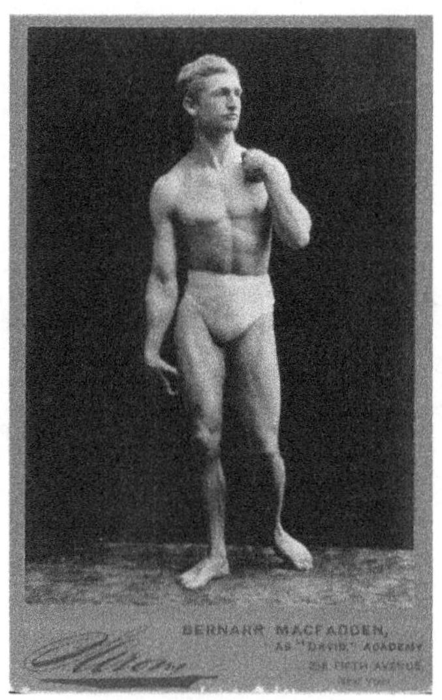

PLATE 4.5. Bernarr MacFadden, publisher of *Physical Culture Magazine* and twentieth century fitness guru, Cabinet card (1900). Courtesy of The Magazine Archives, San Francisco.

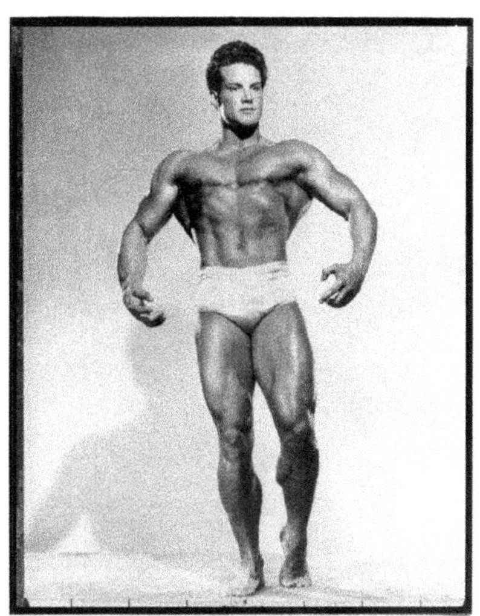

PLATE 4.6. Steve Reeves, Mr. America 1947, and first bodybuilder to become a movie star, photographer unknown (1940s). Courtesy of The Magazine Archives, San Francisco.

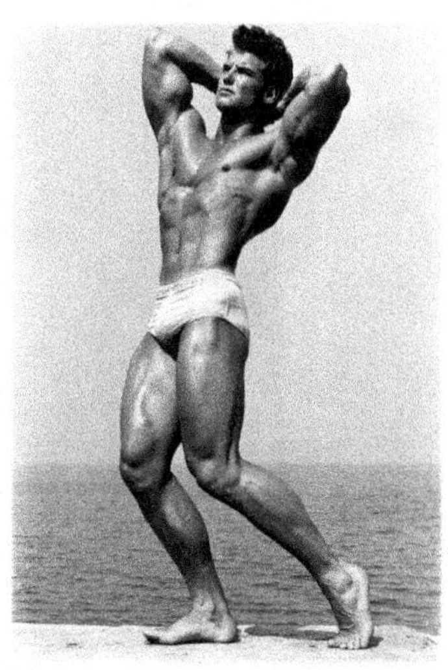

PLATE 4.7. Steve Reeves, Mr. America 1947, taken on the Chicago waterfront by Tony Lanza of Montreal (1940s). Courtesy of The Magazine Archives, San Francisco.

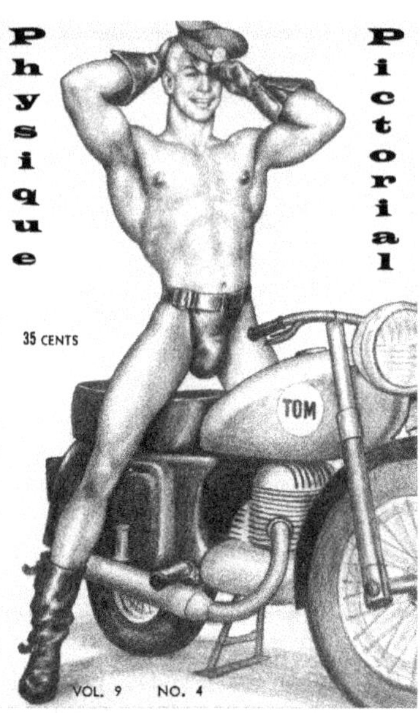

PLATE 4.8. Physique Pictorial cover by Tom of Finland, Volume 9, No. 4 (1960). Courtesy of AthleticModelGuild.com.

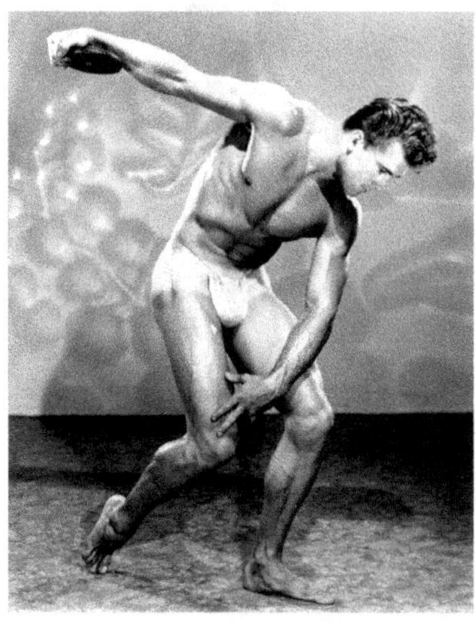

PLATE 4.9. Ed Fury, physique model, by Bob Mizer (1950s). Courtesy of AthleticModelGuild.com.

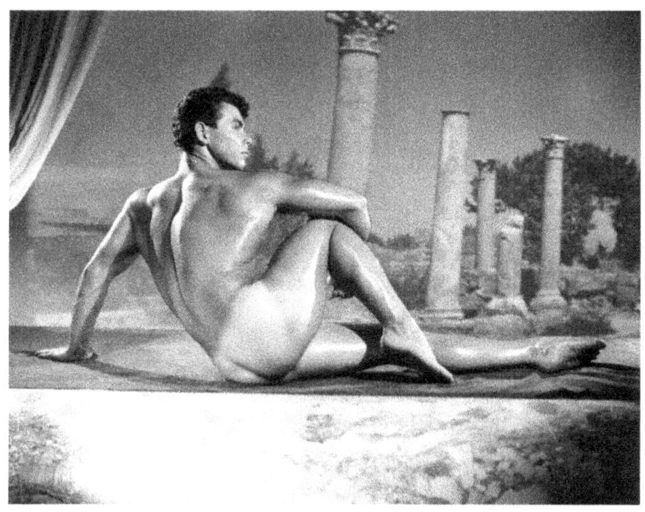

PLATE 4.10. Unidentified physique model, by Bob Mizer (1950s). Courtesy of AthleticModelGuild.com.

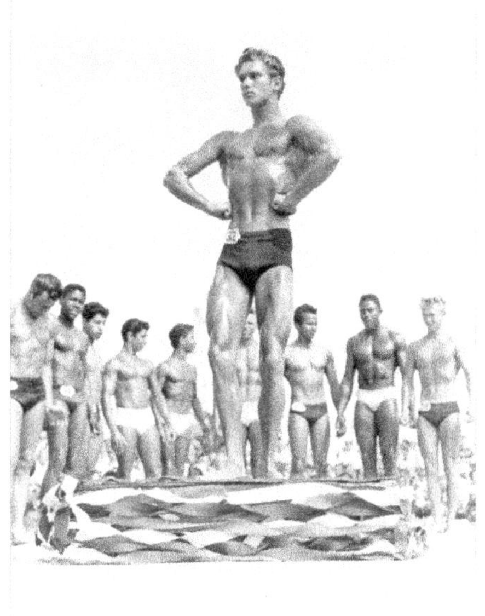

PLATE 4.11. Unidentified contestant at a Muscle Beach physique competition, by Bob Mizer (1940s). Courtesy of AthleticModelGuild.com.

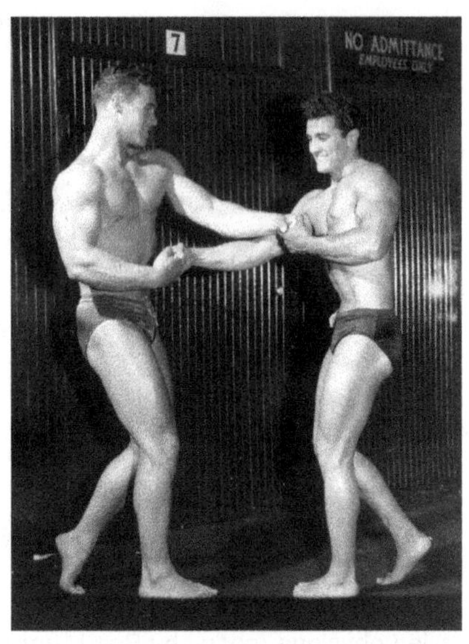

PLATE 4.12. Unidentified bodybuilders, by Bob Mizer (1940s). Courtesy of AthleticModelGuild.com.

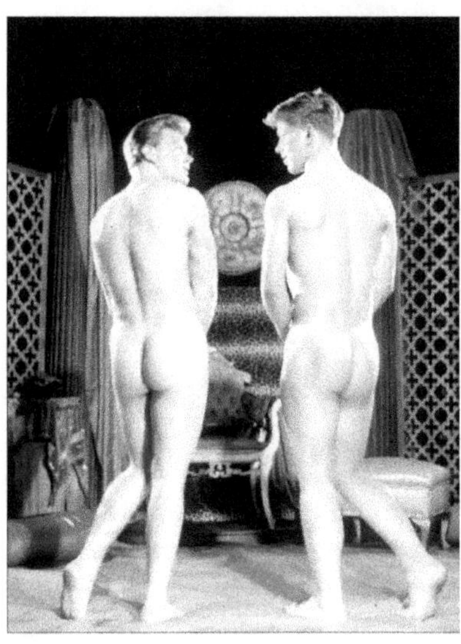

PLATE 4.13. Bill and Nolan, physique models, by Bob Mizer (1950s). Courtesy of AthleticModelGuild.com.

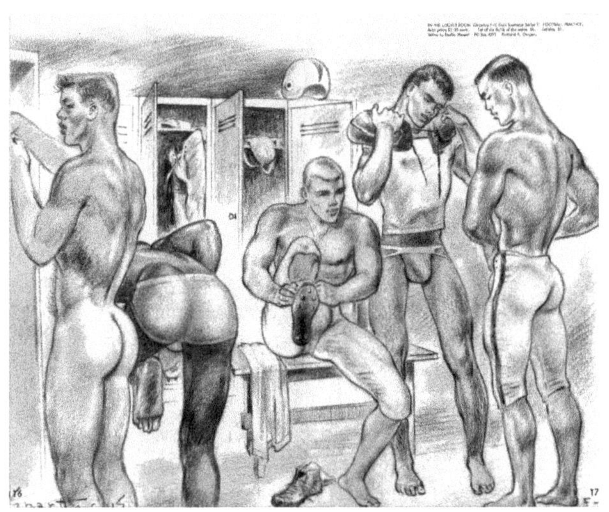

PLATE 4.14. "In the Locker Room" drawing from Spartacus Series F "Football Practice," featured in Physique Pictorial Volume 01, Number 09 (1951). Courtesy of AthleticModelGuild.com.

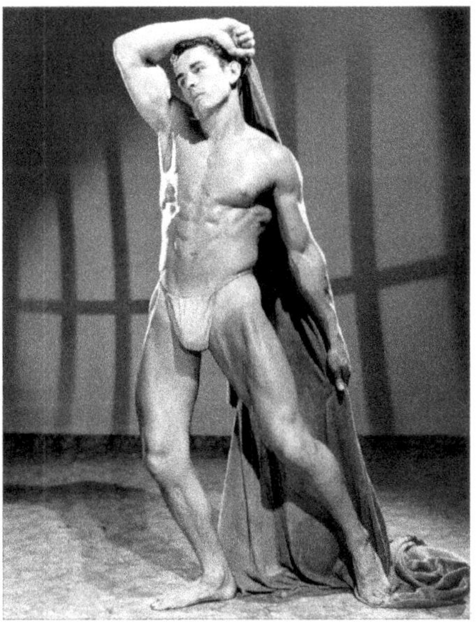

PLATE 4.15. Leonard Chambers, physique model, by Bob Mizer (1950s). Courtesy of AthleticModelGuild.com.

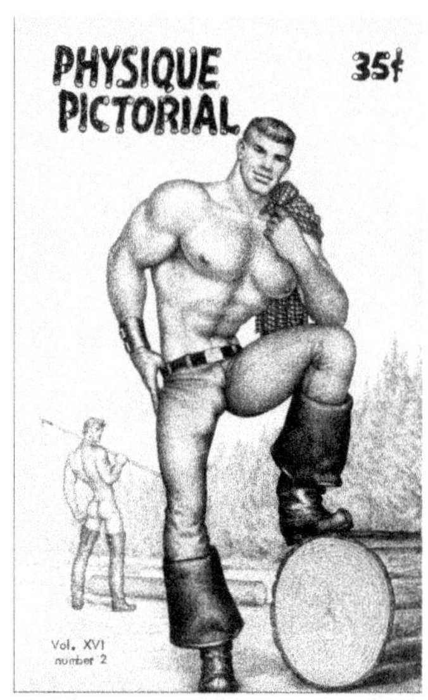

PLATE 4.16. Physique Pictorial cover by Tom of Finland, volume 16, number 2 (1967). Courtesy of AthleticModelGuild.com.

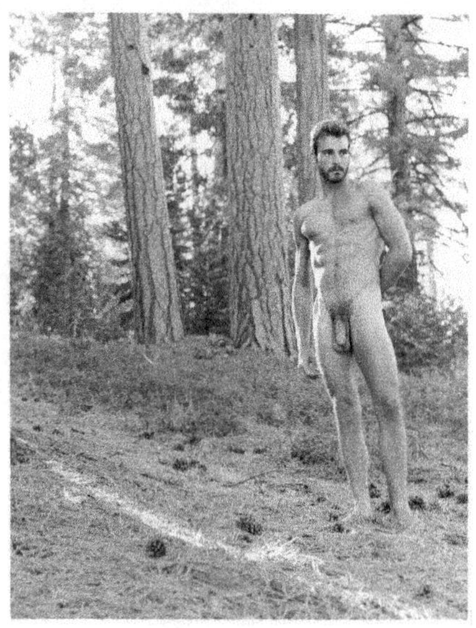

PLATE 4.17. Al Parker, 1970's porn star and famous "clone," by Jim French (1970s). Courtesy of ColtStudio.com.

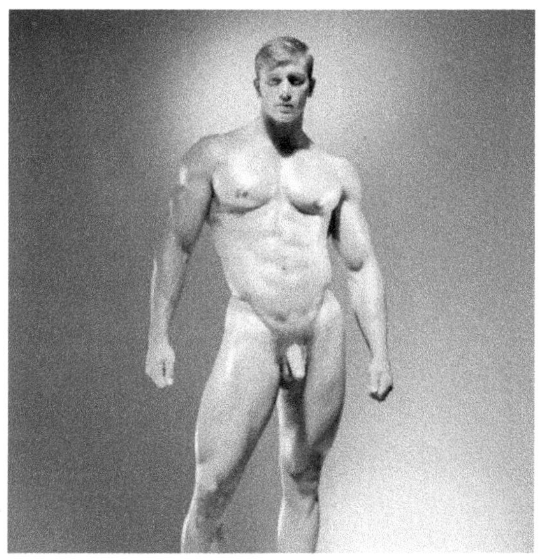

PLATE 4.18. John Pruitt, porn star, by Jim French (1980s). Courtesy of ColtStudio.com.

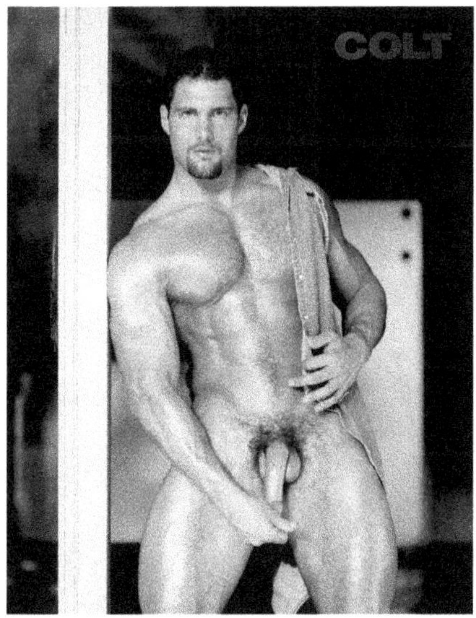

PLATE 4.19. Franco Corelli, porn star, by Jim French (1990s). Courtesy of ColtStudio.com.

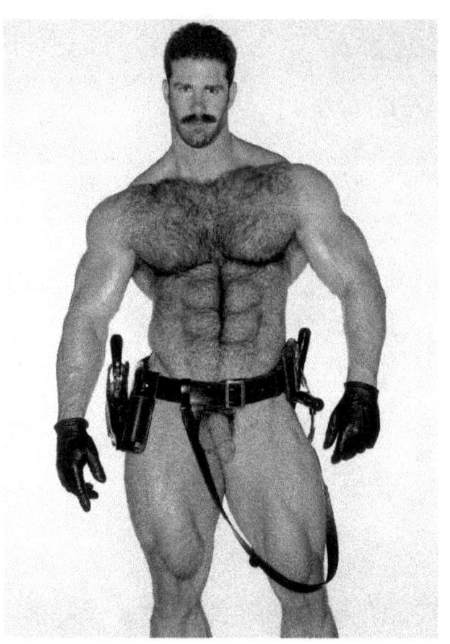

PLATE 4.20. Pete Kuzak, porn star, by Jim French (2000s). Courtesy of ColtStudio.com.

Chapter 7

The Poz Jock

Robert Wallace

After graduating from Harvard Law School, Robert Wallace (a pseudonym) moved to New York, where, by twenty-nine, he had become a successful lawyer. For the boy who had grown up in a small town in Indiana, life seemed picture perfect. Then one Saturday morning, which he remembers like it was yesterday, Robert went down to the lobby of his Manhattan apartment building to get the paper, and he read a *The New York Times* headline that terrified him: "Rare cancer affects gay men."[1] It was July 3, 1981. Standing in the lobby, reading the article, he recalled a muggy day in the summer of 1979 when his lymph nodes had swollen enormously and he felt extremely ill and fatigued. Alarmed, he had gone to his doctor, who confirmed that in fact something was terribly wrong. The doctor had said, "I have no idea what it is; I've never seen anything like it." Robert's symptoms went away, and life went back to normal—for a while. Then that morning came when he stood there reading and all he could think was, "I'm going to die."[2] A mind-numbing wait became the focus of his attention: for the next ten years, every morning after waking up he wondered if that was the day that he would become sick.

In 1982 it was confirmed: he tested positive for HIV. Terrified, he did not have sex for the next two years. He remained healthy for five years, but the virus was slowly destroying his immune system. Robert started getting sick. It was 1987, the negative stigma surrounding AIDS kept him from telling his employer, and there were no effective treatments yet. Robert's life had changed dramatically. It became common for one of his friends to come down with *Pneumocystis carinii* pneumonia (PCP) and to die over the weekend. He also remem-

Muscle Boys: Gay Gym Culture
Published by The Haworth Press, Taylor & Francis Group, 2008.
doi:10.1300/6034_07

bers how, quite often, the person standing next him on the subway was covered in horrendous Kaposi's sarcoma (KS) lesions.

After picking up Bernie S. Siegel's *Love, Medicine, and Miracles,* an exceptional mind-body self-healing book, Robert made some lifestyle changes and decided that he was not going to run for the subway car any longer. "I had to put my well-being first, before my work, other people's expectations, or anything else." His health improved slightly, and it started to look like he would survive the next few years.

But by 1996, Robert's body could no longer fight the HIV: his T-cells (the body's white blood cells that fight infections) were dropping fast, and his viral load was rising even faster. Fortunately, highly active antiretroviral therapies (HAART) had just been introduced, and he started treatment right away. The side effects of the toxic treatment made him feel worse than he ever had from the virus, the diarrhea was nonstop, and his fatigue was incapacitating. By early 1997 he had lost most of his body fat, so much that his pants would fall down. Robert's body was wasting, and he became extremely depressed.

AIDS AND WASTING

The connection between AIDS wasting syndrome, anabolic steroids, and gay gym culture dates to the beginning of the epidemic, which violently attacked the gay community in the early- to mid-1980s. At the time, the untreatable and most physical signs of the disease such as KS and wasting syndrome would clearly mark those who were infected. "Wasting," defined as involuntary loss of more than 10 percent of baseline body weight, is caused by fatigue, diarrhea, and loss of appetite and occurs usually because of an infection due to the underlying HIV disease. It was such a common feature of AIDS that it soon became an AIDS-defining illness. Wasting, it became clear, was one of the most threatening features of AIDS, for as the wasting transpired, the loss of protein occurred not only in the muscles but also in the organs, making them unable to function, eventually taking the life of the person infected.

Alex Cabot (a pseudonym), a retired architect who, at the height of the epidemic, was in his twenties and living in San Francisco, remembers watching his friends and acquaintances transform from "strong, virile, gorgeous young men at the prime of their lives into evaporated, shriveled, walking scarecrows in a matter of weeks." He recalls that the changes occurred so fast and were so drastic that sometimes "you wouldn't recognize your own friends." Feeling angry, outraged, and afraid of who was going to be next, he would at times burst into tears at just the sight of someone with the wasting syndrome.[3]

Having become one of the most threatening features associated with the disease, fighting wasting in patients with AIDS and HIV became a crucial challenge for the medical community. According to Lawrence Price, MD, an HIV specialist in San Francisco, research in the 1980s that was based on body composition analysis and survival factors established that it was the loss of lean muscle mass that proved fatal. Increasing lean mass at any cost was an ideal and extremely valuable element of treatment and prevention of AIDS. As a consequence, anabolic steroids entered the picture.[4]

In the summer of 1998, emaciated and somewhat hopeless, Robert placed a desperate call to his doctor, who prescribed to him synthetic testosterone and Deca Durabolin, both anabolic steroids. He made Robert promise that he would work out hard, and Robert followed his doctor's advice unbendingly. By winter of that same year, he began to feel as if he was getting his life back, that his body "was not a wasted shell." His body responded to the cocktail and to the steroids. After receiving his new lease on life, he moved to San Francisco. His health improved dramatically, and recent test results show an undetectable viral load and T-cells at a twenty-year high.

Robert is one of my clients; he trains hard, eats healthy, takes vitamins and supplements, and doesn't abuse his body. He's no longer depressed and leads a full life. I feel exceptionally lucky to know him; he's one of the happiest men I know. His once-failing body has over the past few years grown to bodybuilder proportions, and a few weeks ago he told me that we should go into a maintenance mode, as he doesn't really want to get any bigger or more muscular. Now, the fifty-two-year-old is often pursued by men twenty or thirty years younger than he, men who find themselves in awe of his unpretentious personality and of course, his beautiful body. When asked about his self-image and how he feels about his body now, Robert's blue eyes glint, he smiles, and he sums it all up in one word: "fabulous."

Robert's story is surely one of a man overcoming adversity. But it also tells the story of how an unfortunate situation created a new and influential subculture in gay gym and body culture—the "poz jock"—a new type of athlete, a gym-sort-of-jock who must adhere to his workouts and his diet with just as much vigilance and with a hell of a lot more at stake than a professional athlete. This chapter tells their story.

THE ANABOLIC STEROID SOLUTION

Testosterone is the natural male hormone. Although it is present in women as well in small amounts, its concentration is much higher in men—by a ratio of 20 to 1. Anabolic steroids are a group of man-made, testosterone-like hormones. Scientists in Europe first synthesized them in the 1930s to treat hypogonadism, a hormonal imbalance in which the testes do not produce enough testosterone. In young men, low testosterone levels can interfere with normal growth and development. In adult males, it can affect energy, sexual function, and desire. Hypogonadism is common in HIV-positive men and can result in muscle wasting. Occasionally, it occurs in HIV-negative men over forty.

Body composition is a critical component in the management of HIV and AIDS, and because of anabolic steroids' effectiveness in building muscle, they are being used more and more in patients with HIV and AIDS. Anabolic steroids were used before the now-popular HAART; these days, they're often used in combination with HAART for treatment and prevention. As treatment, they are more commonly used for hypogonadism. As a prevention tool, they build a reserve of lean mass in case the patient comes down with PCP or an opportunistic infection and loses twenty or thirty pounds.

In a telephone interview from his home in West Hollywood, California, Michael Mooney, co-author of the highly acclaimed book on anabolic steroids and HIV, *Built to Survive,* explained to me that anabolic steroids are valuable to HIV-positive men because not only do these men continually show low testosterone levels but they are also confronted with a compromised immune system. He explains that because of the stress that HIV places on the body and because of a number of other problems such as insulin or testosterone resistance, the testosterone doses required for HIV-positive men are about twice as high as the normal 100-milligram-a-week doses that are normally prescribed to HIV-negative men with hypogonadism. Mooney also emphasized that for anabolic steroids to work optimally, the person using them needs not only to follow an aggressive exercise routine, but also eat a high protein diet.[5]

Mooney also mentioned the importance of steroids in managing lipodystrophy, which is commonly seen in patients on HAART therapy. Lipodystrophy refers to the accumulated fat deposits that show up in the abdominal area known as "protease pouch" or at the back of the neck known as "buffalo hump." Because of the muscle-building and fat-burning effects that steroids have, the fat deposits can be reversed to some extent with anabolic therapy. On the other hand, too much of a fat-burning effect can result in a less desirable feature in which the use of steroids can increase facial wasting. This fat-loss effect is not as radical as what has been associated with the anti-HIV medication Zerit (D4T), but it can be significant. Facial wasting is a component of the lipodystrophy set of symptoms, characterized by sunken cheeks from the loss of the thin layer of fat under the skin of the face. Facial wasting doesn't pose a health risk, but is more and more becoming an identifying feature among those HIV-positive men on HAART therapy and/or steroids; it represents yet another emotional and social burden on the patient. In addition, Mooney points out the benefits of steroids as treatment for depression and what he calls the "psychological impotence" that HIV-positive men can face, often with the result of "getting depressed men off the couch and into the gym, or back to work."[6]

Lennart Moller, MD, a specialist in HIV psychiatry in San Francisco, told me that physicians initially prescribed steroids only to patients who showed signs of wasting. But they now prescribe anabolic steroids to many HIV-positive men. Moller noted that wasting affects not only outer muscles, but also internal organs, which can lead to organ failure and death. Steroids also give patients more energy, better appetite, and improved mood, he said. "It started out specifically for people who had a lot of weight loss due to AIDS and from there, over the years in the early nineties, they started being prescribed more and more."[7]

Although there are many different types of anabolic steroids, the most commonly used are synthetic testosterone, Deca Durabolin, and human growth hormone. Depending on the steroid, they may be taken orally, intramuscularly, or through recently introduced testosterone skin and scrotal patches or gel. In HIV-positive or hypogonadal men on testosterone therapy, the gel and the patches are applied daily; these seem to be easier to manage, as the level of testosterone in the body remains constant. With the weekly or biweekly injections, men are more susceptible to experience a roller coaster of energy, emotions, and aggressiveness. As Moller explains, "Once you get above the doses that are usually in the body, testosterone can cause increasing amounts of aggressiveness in a person and this can lead to arguments, road rage, fights, and a lot of interpersonal difficulties."[8]

It's almost impossible to estimate the percentage of HIV-positive men on the anabolic therapies. Although some physicians calculate that 5 percent or less of their patients are on the drugs, others estimate that up to 60 percent of their HIV-positive patients are on them. What it comes down to is how the physician feels about anabolic steroids and, to a great degree, where the patient lives. Doctors in large metropolitan areas are more likely to prescribe the controversial drugs to their patients.

Of course, taking steroids is only part of the therapy: for the drugs to work optimally, patients need, most of all, to eat accordingly and pump iron.

SURVIVAL OF THE BUFFEST

Because of steroid treatment, in the 1980s the AIDS epidemic sent into the gym thousands and thousands of HIV-positive gay men who previously had no interest in lifting weights and exercising, let alone bodybuilding. In a strange twist of fate, the frail and weak would build themselves into rock-solid, strong men, assembling a small army of bodybuilders never before seen as a sizeable contingent of gay culture. The medical benefits of anabolic steroids became invaluable; those taking them not only improved their health and quality of life, but also soon reported an immense boost to their deteriorating self-image. Before long they were being noticed and admired by other men, desirable once again, sometimes more than ever.

Ron Tripp, a personal trainer in San Francisco who has been positive since 1986 and is on anabolic therapy, reports that not only does he feel better when a bio impedance analysis (a body composition test) shows a higher percent of lean mass, but his blood tests come back with superior numbers. Tripp's self-image has also improved as a result of the anabolic therapy: "It makes me feel more secure, more comfortable, more masculine, and more confident socially and sexually." He also notes that he has more energy, thinks better, and his sex drive is higher. The only shortcomings, he says, are that "I sweat more, feel more aggressive and a little less patient."[9]

But the steroid prescriptions led to a new controversy in the gay gym community. On one hand, men in the community who were HIV negative felt a sense of desire troubled by fear toward these men, for they represented an ideal of male beauty yet they carried risk of infection. On the other hand, HIV-negative men felt resentful not only of the easy access to which the HIV-positive men could get a prescription for steroids, but also of the time that those who were on Disability (and not working) could spend at the gym. Insensitive to the price at which the gym-built body came, it was not long before one could hear the double-edged acronym describing them as *GODS* (Gays on Disability and Steroids).

Ron Tripp is well aware of the tension and explains that he has many times experienced "attitude from HIV [negative] men who are bothered about the fact that HIV-positive men who were frail, weaker, and gaunt are now more muscular, bigger, and stronger than they are." [10]Feeling that they could not compete at the gym or in the buff without using steroids themselves, more and more men began using the drugs, which are easily obtainable via the black market at most gyms. This situation has generated a domino effect in gay gym culture as more and more men, positive or negative, are using or want to use the magic drugs. Because he is a personal trainer and people are aware of both his HIV status and the steroids, people at the gym approach Tripp almost weekly—friends and friends of friends who ask him to get steroids for them. Professionally and politely, he tells them to consult their doctor first and warns them of the danger in buying second-hand steroids from the street.

RISKS AND BENEFITS

Depending on the individual's body type, fitness starting point, and metabolism, the use of anabolic steroids almost always results in muscle growth (hypertrophy), decreased body fat, increased strength, increased training tolerance (greater intensity, faster recovery), increased sex drive, and in some cases even hyperplasia, the multiplication of muscle cells, which normally stops occurring when boys reach puberty. Although most of these results are desirable for most men interested in fitness or sports, and for obvious aesthetic reasons, the use of anabolic steroids nevertheless comes with possible health risks as well as the negative social stigma associated with them.

Although the most common negative side effects with anabolic steroids are oily skin, acne, and aggressiveness, there are also a number of health risks associated with their long-term use and most significantly when the drugs are abused. When they are used for a long period of time, especially at high doses, the numerous side effects can include heart disease, liver problems, prostate enlargement, irritability, and increased aggressiveness. It should be noted that while most athletes and bodybuilders who use anabolics typically take about twice the prescribed dose, people who abuse them have been known to take ten to forty times the clinical therapeutic doses—at these levels, manic and psychotic episodes, not to mention an exponential presence of risk factors, are easily explainable.[11] The long-term use of human growth hormone can also cause acromegaly, the elongating and enlargement of bones of the extremities and certain bones of the head, especially the frontal bone and the jaws.[12] For those not under the supervision of a medical doctor, aside from the physical negative side effects, come the possible social and legal drawbacks of using a controlled substance.

The biggest problems and risks associated with anabolic steroids, from a medical perspective, surface when the drugs are abused. Another San Francisco doctor (who wishes to remain anonymous) recalls an HIV-positive patient (I'll call him Tom) who asked for an anabolic steroid prescription; because his T-cells and testosterone levels were low and the patient was concerned about wasting, the physician wrote the script. After a few weeks, the patient's blood tests revealed diabetes and dangerously high blood pressure, cholesterol and sugar levels. Because he had gained so much muscle mass, the doctor questioned whether he was taking more than the prescribed amount of the anabolics. "Tom" admitted that he had been buying additional amounts of both testosterone and Deca Durabolin on the black market and taking several times his prescribed dose. Alarmed, the physician instructed him to immediately get off the higher underground dose, which he had not prescribed.Tom refused. After only two months, Tom came back to the hospital. This time it wasn't so pleasant—he had suffered a mild stroke as a result of abusing steroids. He recovered from the stroke and hoped to get back on the steroids, but the doctor refused to prescribe them. Tom found another physician who was willing to prescribe them, and is on the drugs again.

Lennart Moller is familiar with the problem many doctors come across when working with HIV-positive patients:

> Prescribing testosterone to people with AIDS and HIV was definitely a needed thing. I mean, people would have died. But in the mid to late 1990s it became overly prescribed. I think a lot of it was mostly patient driven: people would see their friends who were looking on death's door and were prescribed anabolic steroids and six months later, they were working out, and looked fabulous. Even the guys who didn't have the weight loss were going in and one way or another—maybe pressuring or not quite being honest with their doctor—would get prescribed testosterone.[13]

Part of the problem for a physician in prescribing anabolic steroids, specifically testosterone, the most popular one, is that the range of what is "normal" in a patient is very broad. A blood test can measure a person's testosterone and assign a value within a range; the problem with this test is that the normal range is between 300 and 1,200. "It is completely inexact science, and very hard to say for sure what a person's level probably is or should be," Moller says.

To complicate matters, Moller tells me, testosterone is in some ways similar to insulin. The puzzle surrounding testosterone-deficient symptoms is similar to adult-onset diabetes, which occurs when body cells become resistant to insulin and do not respond to the hormone. When this happens, "even though the person may have really high levels of insulin in their [*sic*] blood stream, their body is just not responding to it like it should and it's very possible that a similar faulty mechanism can occur with other hormones [such as testosterone] in the body."[14]

Unlike insulin however, testosterone research is very limited for the sole reason that studying it can get you thrown in jail

THE LAW AND THE BLACK MARKET

Anabolic steroids were legal by prescription in the United States even for cosmetic purposes until the fall of 1990, when Congress passed the Anabolic Steroid Act. According to the U.S. Drug Enforcement Administration (DEA), the law, which became effective in 1991, classified twenty-seven steroids as Schedule III substances under the Controlled Substances Act. Later, the Anabolic Steroid Control Act of 2004 added an additional thirty-two steroids in Schedule III and expanded the DEA's "regulatory and enforcement authority regarding steroids."[15] Although steroids are legal in many other countries, in the United States it is now illegal to possess or distribute anabolic steroids without a prescription under federal and state laws. Physicians can prescribe anabolic steroids for certain conditions such as hypogonadism and wasting. Under current laws, and these vary by state, the possession of nonprescribed anabolic steroids is a federal offense that can be punishable by up to one year in prison and a minimum fine of $1,000 for simple possession or up to five years in prison and a fine of $250,000 for possession with intent to sell.

The criminalization of anabolic steroids naturally resulted in an increase in the underground black market. The DEA Web site notes that following the enactment of the Anabolic Steroid Control Act, "street prices of anabolic steroids have increased substantially as a result." Depending on the source and the specific drugs, the street price of the average six- to twelve-week steroid cycle runs about $500. Meanwhile, the National Institute on Drug Abuse (NIDA) in 1997 reported that the dollar value of the black market had reached an estimated $400 million.[16] Neither the DEA nor the NIDA had updated this figure by 2006, but experts on anabolic steroids, believe that dollar amount to be greatly underestimated. Because anabolic steroids are legal in Mexico and Europe, they can easily be mailed to the United States, making it "impossible to attack the trafficking at its source," notes the DEA.

In the gay community, where many disabled men with AIDS live under impoverished conditions and are trying to survive on insufficient Disability and Social Security payments, there is yet another dimension to the black market of anabolic steroids. Like destitute senior citizens selling their Vicodin or Valium on the streets to make ends meet, HIV-positive men are selling their steroids in gay urban America. The large and growing market of HIV-negative gay men who want to take the drugs and the vast number of underprivileged people with AIDS make this equation a no-brainer.

Contributing to the black market is the accessibility to anabolic steroids available on the Internet. Because the drugs can be prescribed, it is possible to find a physician that will prescribe them if the patient claims certain symptoms through an online or telephone consultation (typically, symptoms associated with hypogonadism). There are, of course, serious side effects to an online prescription. For one, the purity of the drugs is questionable, and from the warnings on most bulletin boards of steroid community's Web sites, it seems that people looking to get their muscles ripped are only getting their wallets ripped off. For another, your "doctor" can turn out to be an undercover cop.

Criminalization of the drugs creates another problem for HIV-positive men. Because they are a controlled substance, physicians may be reluctant to prescribe them, even when the patient really needs them. Eddie Winslow (a pseudonym), a thirty-five-year-old, Boston-based personal trainer and longtime HIV-positive survivor, who is well versed in anabolic therapy, has not been able to receive a testosterone prescription from his doctor even though his levels are very low, he has lost about twenty pounds, and has very little energy. Eddie has been asking his physician for three years, and despite all of the medical research and evidence on the matter, the doctor flat out refuses.

THE AESTHETIC DEBATE

Anabolic steroids are sought after because they work. When combined with a high-intensity exercise program, a high-calorie and high-protein diet, and adequate rest, they can promote muscle growth and strength beyond one's normal capacity. They are typically taken in six- to twelve-week cycles, and after the cycle is over, some, though not all, of the muscle mass gained is maintained. Most athletes who use them do one or two cycles a year. Staying on the drugs continuously—and many people do this—is abusing them.

A great number of people seem to have strong convictions against them because of the unconstructive sensationalism that has been generated by the media. Although not entirely, the majority of the media's "big stories" concern the controversy in competitive sports, where steroids are banned for the simple reason that they provide a real physiological advantage to athletes. The biggest fault by the media is that more often than not, they fail to cover a story properly when it comes to steroids. More specifically, many journalists fail to make clear that their stories have arisen out of steroid *abuse—not steroid use.*

Jason Six (a pseudonym) is a thirty-four-year-old HIV-positive man who lives in Los Angeles. Like most people, Jason's reaction to steroids was based on the lack of education. "I didn't know anyone who had done them at the time," he said.[17] "I had the type of mentality that most people do: it's scary, it's a needle, you're going to get cancer, et cetera." Then, Jason met another young man with whom he had a brief affair who exposed him to steroid use. "He gave me straight talk about it, told me about using them properly, and the importance of not abusing them. That all you need to do is one cycle a year, get your gains and then stop." Jason brought it up with his doctor, who agreed, and Jason started getting shots every two weeks. Jason's boyfriend wanted to try the drugs, too, and Jason hooked him up by supplying him the drugs from his own prescriptions.

Although in athletic competitions, using steroids gives an unfair advantage and is most definitely unethical, the negative hype around steroid use in noncompetitive athletes is, for the most part, blown out of proportion and the result of inexpert judgment. It was in large part the controversy over ethics in the Olympics that led to the criminalization of steroids. Another major influential concern involves teenage boys taking them in high school to grow more muscular. Because of sports ethics and the risk that steroid abuse can pose to undeveloped youths, conventional wisdom would tell us that having anabolic steroids regulated and under control is the best choice. But to classify anabolic steroids in the same category with heroin, amphetamines, and cocaine only creates criminals out of athletes who typically live responsible, productive lives—very different from those of your typical heroin addict.

Many recreational athletes and bodybuilders make the valid argument that given the microscopic fraction of athletes who actually compete in the Olympics or the Gay Games, the validity of the law is questionable. Because recreational athletes are not going to compete at an elite or professional level, they feel they should be free to maximize their bodies' potential in a safe and sound environment.

Of the 5,576 men who completed my survey, 8.4 percent cite AIDS and HIV management as one of the reasons that they work out and exercise (see Figure 6.2). Yet, in my interviews I came across many HIV-positive men who work out, yet do not cite their HIV status in having anything to do with their exercise regimens. In the United States, HIV and AIDS are now managed quite well with medications, and wasting syndrome is rarely a threat to those infected.

Steroid use in the gay community today has, for the most part, limited relevance to health management; the drugs are largely consumed in an aesthetic-enhancement effort. Of those surveyed, 28 percent or 1,316 men reported having used anabolic steroids; less than half of them (529) had a prescription (see Figure 7.1). It should be noted, however, that because my survey was conducted worldwide, many of the respondents live in countries where the drugs are sold over the counter and as easy to get as a pack of Marlboros. In the United States, prescriptions for anabolic substances are more difficult—yet not impossible—to get, regardless of medical guidelines. As Jason Six's story demonstrates, doctors sometimes prescribe the drugs without much need for persuasion. For others, like his boyfriend, your boyfriend can get them for you. Given the popularity of steroids,

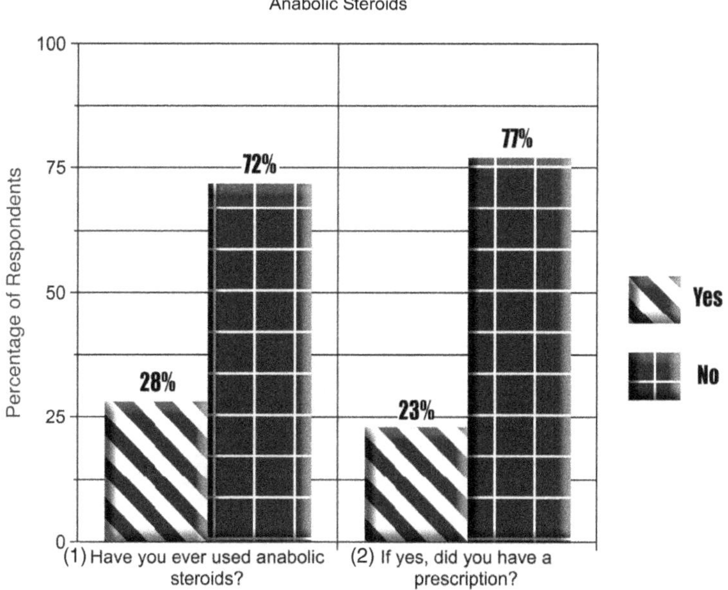

FIGURE 7.1. Anabolic steroids: (1) Prevalence of anabolic steroid use within gay gym culture. (2) Comparison between anabolic steroids obtained by prescription versus obtained illegally.

this is not a difficult task. Seventy percent of the men who completed the survey said that they knew someone who had used anabolic steroids, and when I asked the question "Would you consider using anabolic steroids in the future?" 32 percent said "Yes," and 14 percent said "maybe" (see Figure 7.2).

Yet attitudes about steroid use *for cosmetic reasons* are diverse. In fact, the only other topic discussed in my survey that generated such different answers was sex in the locker room, but we'll get to that later. When asked: "In general how do you feel about men who use anabolic steroids for cosmetic reasons?" 21 percent of respondents reported their use for cosmetic purposes is "OK," and 26 percent felt it is "not OK," yet the majority of respondents, a whopping 52 percent, answered that they felt steroid use is "a personal decision" (see Figure 7.3).

From those who elaborated on their answers, I received some interesting notes: A twenty-five-year-old college student in Canada who

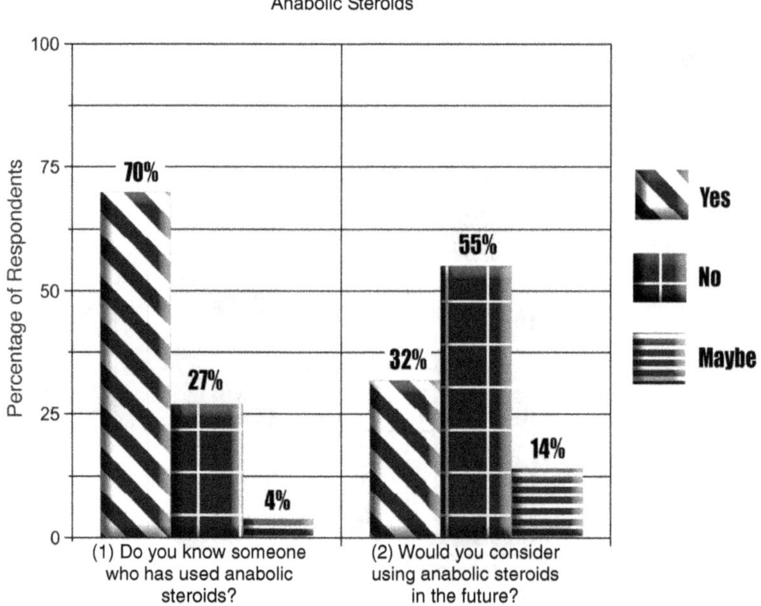

FIGURE 7.2. Anabolic steroids: (1) Percentage of gay gym culture familiar with someone who has used anabolic steroids. (2) Percentage of gay gym culture that would consider or refuse to take anabolic steroids in the future.

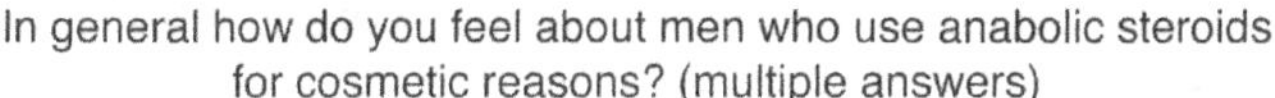

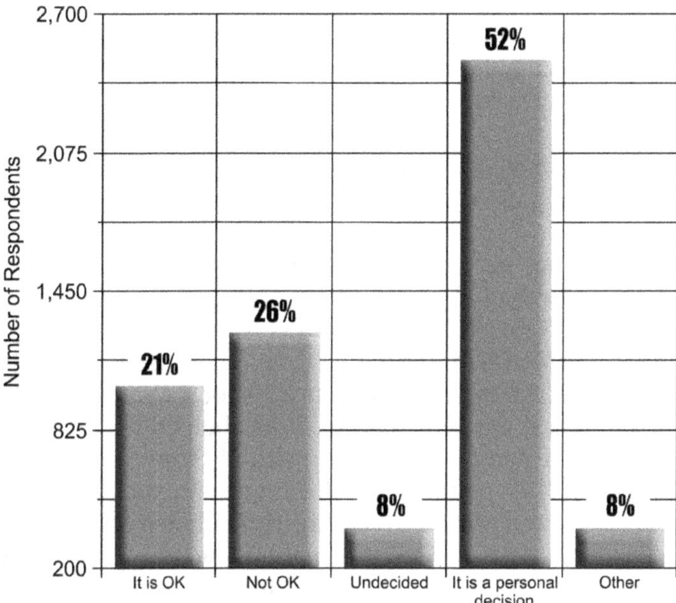

FIGURE 7.3. Different points of view concerning the use of anabolic steroids for cosmetic purposes.

has used steroids without a prescription wrote, "I find it very sexy!" Another college student, a twenty-three-year-old self-described jock, has not used the drugs and thinks that those who use them are "pussies." And a thirty-seven-year-old who identifies as a Bear/Muscle Bear just wanted to know: "How do I get a script?"

A few thought out their answers a little more, but in general their responses were divisive and in disagreement with one another. A twenty-nine-year-old white-collar professional who has used steroids without a prescription and who also indicated that he would use them in the future wrote:

> I feel that it is a personal decision that like EVERYTHING should be used responsibly. For example, when I did try them, my doctor monitored my health closely.

And a fifty-one-year-old from Macon, Georgia, who identifies as a Muscle Bear said:

> I think it is sick, actually. It's so obvious when somebody does it. The look is exaggerated and not attractive. And as soon as you grab their balls you know they are on them.

An HIV-negative, forty-one-year-old from Florida, offered yet another interesting perspective on his use of steroids:

> I view doing steroids the same as cosmetic surgery. It is a very serious, personal decision that should not be chosen on a whim nor done to excess. For me, the decision to use steroids was one that I wrestled with for a long time. I have never done ANY illicit drugs. After talking with my doctor, I chose to do it. I wish I had done it ten years earlier. It has helped me erase much of a very bad body image that resulted from being very small (5-foot-9, 140 pounds) and from some sexual abuse between ages eight and ten. It is NOT the right choice for everyone. For me it was. The increased social and sexual attention was remarkable and unexpected. I feel more confident about myself whether I am at the beach or in a suit for work. People respond to a muscular man with increased attention and intrigue. Socially, I now have social and sexual access to the guys I always fantasized about. I no longer see myself as the skinny, 140-pound weakling.

Many others reiterated the ambiguity about the "magic potions." This thought came from a forty-two-year-old in New York: "It's a personal decision, but one often wrapped in what I see as a lack of self-image and a need to conform to falsely imposed standards of male beauty." This quote is from a forty-three-year-old in New Jersey: "I have mixed feelings about it. For the most part they look great, but since I don't do them, it tends to make me feel inferior." And these feelings from a thirty-eight-year-old in Chicago: "Sad/disappointed, with a tinge of jealousy in terms of results; but never think it's worth it to do myself."

When I discussed the type of debate that goes on among gay men in regard to steroid use for cosmetic purposes with Dr. Lennart

Moller, he basically told me that the medical community debates the issue just as much:

> If you were to go to the AMA [American Medical Association] they would put steroids in the same category as illegal drug abuse and be very much against it. But some doctors feel that if something works for a person and doesn't have a lot of negative consequences maybe it's not such a bad thing. I mean, helping the patient is what we need to be doing and should be doing.[18]

TO JUICE OR NOT TO JUICE?

A couple of years ago I attended a cocktail party in West Hollywood, where everyone quickly noticed "Mark," a beautiful and brawny Italian who, nearly everyone at the party agreed, was the hottest guy there. After a couple of vodka sodas, I built up the courage to excuse myself from my drooling friends and headed to the kitchen for a refill at the same time the Italian jock did. Reaching in the ice bucket at the same time, we cordially introduced ourselves and started talking. As I got closer, not only did I realize that he was more beautiful up close, but that he was smart, charming, and almost sexier than Brad Pitt in *Fight Club.* After I mentioned my work on this book, Mark confided in me that he had been really interested in using steroids. He said that he felt conflicted in between the possible negative side effects and the superficial reasons why he wanted to do them. This being Los Angeles, the dilemma had become one of the main topics discussed between him and his therapist. He added that after a little research, he had even managed to find a doctor on the Internet who would prescribe him the anabolics even though he was HIV negative and had a normal testosterone level. But after some careful consideration he decided to "wait a while." In the following chapters, I discuss in detail the role of steroids in relationship to body image. In the era of "bigger is better," using steroids is tempting for any man—even in the case of Mark, who, by general consensus, did not need to change a thing.

Men who are pondering the question "To juice or not to juice?" *for cosmetic reasons* should educate themselves on the subject matter and consider the following before making a decision.

First, although they are highly efficient, anabolic steroids are not as magical as they seem. To see results, you have to do a lot of the hard work yourself. This requires extreme amounts of discipline, time, and energy dedicated to training at advanced levels; following a fairly strict diet that involves a lot of planning, cost, and preparation; and more than adequate rest. It's basically a part-time job. The point is, unless you have a metabolic problem, by following the same strategy and going natural, most men under forty can achieve impressive results. Of course it will take longer and you will have to work harder, but the results will also be more permanent.

Second, take into consideration whether you are advanced enough and have truly *peaked* and maximized your body's own natural potential. Most men have not. I've had many clients, known many men at the gym, and have myself achieved the same results in a year's time as other men I've known to be on anabolic steroids.

Third, there's always the risk that unless you're getting steroids from your doctor, their safety and effectiveness are highly questionable. As with any other street drug, unless you are 100 percent sure of the source, you might be getting a less effective, diluted version, or, worse, a fake.

Fourth, considering that the possible health risks involved are unnecessary *and* avoidable—much like those in cosmetic surgery, ask yourself "why"—and honestly examine your answer.

Last, but not least, is the ugly fact that steroids are illegal, and a criminal conviction for possession can result not only in a stay in jail, but it is also ridiculously expensive, emotionally exhausting, and permanently under your weight belt.

As an exercise physiologist and a personal trainer, I often get faced with the questions of whether I am in opposition or in favor of steroids for cosmetic purposes. The truth is, I vacillate. I'm more interested in informing you of the pros and cons without telling you whether they are good or bad, then leaving you to make your own decision. As a person fascinated with the male physique and the body's potential, I'm intrigued. And as a single gay man on such a competitive meat market, who to put it frankly would like to get laid more often, and at human moments feels insecure and oblivious to everything I learned in years of psychotherapy, I get just as tempted as everyone else.

Chapter 8

The Gay Athlete

Scott Robinson is one of San Francisco's most popular athletes. When he's not working, he's training, whether it is for a triathlon, the next AIDS Ride cycling event, or a swimming competition. Born in Texas and raised in Iowa, Scott attended Williams College in western Massachusetts where he studied geology. After college he lived in Virginia and Oregon before settling in San Francisco. But one thing that has been constant in Scott's life is his involvement in sports. He started swimming when he was six and has gone on to coach and compete at semi-professional levels for several years. Along the way he picked up cycling and running, eventually completing several marathons and triathlons while placing respectably in his age group.

Scott has twice completed the California AIDS Ride, a 560-mile cycling fundraiser from San Francisco to Los Angles. He has also twice lived in tents for a month and a half during geology field seasons in Antarctica. He's gone backpacking in New Hampshire, canoeing in Canada, sea kayaking in California, river surfing in New Zealand, mountain biking in Oregon, and cross-country and downhill skiing in Virginia. As part of a relay swim team Scott was instrumental in setting two American records at the Gay Games in Sydney (master's national records in 400-meter and 800-meter freestyle relays).

Sporting a hard and lean body and a handsome yet wholesome face, Scott is the embodiment of the all-American athlete—the classic jock. He is also a gay man. This combination of characteristics caused conflict when he was coming of age:

> My first gay experience was in college. I was a freshman, and it happened in the dorm room after a party, but it freaked me out. We never talked about it, it didn't happen again, and I avoided him after that. Eventually I started dating a guy—we were best

Muscle Boys: Gay Gym Culture
Published by The Haworth Press, Taylor & Francis Group, 2008.
doi:10.1300/6034_08

> friends, he was a cross-country runner, and we were having sex, but we never talked about it. I had couple of experiences like that, and eventually got involved with another guy, another athlete, and again never talked about it even though the relationship went on for about seven years. I always thought I'd find the right woman, was always in denial, never dealt with it. Part of it was because at that time, I had bought into what the media said a gay person was: very flamboyant, very feminine, and that wasn't how I saw myself. I didn't want to be that way. It wasn't until I started meeting these athletic gay people in Virginia and Oregon that I was able to finally come out. I was twenty-nine when I first said, "I am gay."[1]

Much has changed in the decades since Scott Robinson came to terms with being both an athlete and a gay man. There was a change in perception and a deconstruction of the strongly held stereotypes that had for centuries been attached to both the male athlete and the male homosexual, making it virtually impossible for the same man to be both. Athletic organizations such as Frontrunners, the Gay Games, and many others were organized as a response to the conflict, and as a result more and more gay men are pursuing athletics. There is, nevertheless, still a paradoxical association that comes with being a gay athlete, even in gay culture today. In professional sports, with only a few exceptions, homophobia rules the athletic closet.

Twenty-four percent (1,188) of the men who completed my survey identified themselves as "jocks" or "athletes" (see Figure 6.1). Most of these guys, mind you, are not professional athletes; they are recreational athletes. Professional athletes are a fascinating breed to study and write about, but they have been written about quite a bit and they amount to only a tiny percentage of all gym culture. Later we will talk about professional gay athletes. In this chapter the focus is on the guys who shop at the same grocery store as you do—guys like Scott and Raymond—for whom being athletic is a passion and lifestyle rather than a profitable career.

Raymond Pajek is a triathlete who was born in Hollywood and grew up in the San Francisco Bay area. He settled with his partner, another triathlete, in the Oakland Hills east of San Francisco. The forty-two-year-old (who appears ten years younger) has been competing in triathlons for the past fifteen years—he swims, bikes, and runs and is a member of the Walnut Creek Masters swim team. He also hits the gym several times a week (depending on the season) to cross train with weights, and when he does he prefers to work out at a gay gym:

> I prefer a gay gym or one that has a strong gay presence; I think it's one of the few areas of my life where I can feel like I'm part of the gay community. Because I don't live in the Castro now. When I came to San Francisco, the gay gym was kind of an indoctrination into gay culture because I came out shortly after I moved back home from college. So the gay men at the gym became a part of my extended community, and now, maybe 15 years later, I still see some of the same people at the gym—that's why I like it.[2]

In this chapter I examine the place that gay athletes hold in gym culture as well as in athletics. Then, in an effort to understand gay athleticism, I examine the strongly held stereotypes and definitions of both sides of this coin: the gay male and the male athlete. Furthermore, I will take a look at the rapidly growing field of gay athletics and sports that has grown over the past thirty years. Last, I discuss the darkness of the athletic closet of professional sports.

ATHLETES AND THE GYM

In the recent past, many athletes were discouraged from exercising with weights or performing other types of strength-training activities because many coaches erroneously believed that building the muscles would take away from the athletes' specific sport. The theory was that any bodybuilding would reduce the athletes' range of motion or skill in the execution of certain movements. Even as recently as four years ago, when I was training for a triathlon, I had a swim coach tell me to lose some muscle. Like many other exercise-related theories, this is one that has been proved wrong by scientific research in the exercise physiology field.

Exercise physiology is a fairly new field, but what has come out of the scientific research in the past few decades has been of enormous consequence. It has changed the way athletes live, train, and eat. Now, while it's true that excessive amounts of muscle mass could limit an athlete's range of motion, the operative word is *excessive:* for muscle to be limiting to the athlete it must be truly "Incredible Hulk"–

like, not just muscular. In just about every athlete, extra muscle translates into extra strength, power, and even muscular endurance. You build that extra muscle by lifting weights. In addition, weight training increases not just the strength of the muscles but also of the joints, which helps considerably in keeping an athlete injury free or helping him recover from his training much quicker.

The field of exercise physiology has also addressed and is working to change yet another myth about male athletes: the *dumb jock* stereotype. The physical power and aggressiveness often required for sports overshadows the high level of mental capacity necessary to be a successful athlete. It is still common, even today, for the uneducated layperson to be ignorant of the brainpower involved in a skillfully executed movement or game. Fortunately, the dumb jock stereotype is losing ground as athletics become more popular within educated groups of corporate America and academia. Recent studies in neuroscience and kinesiology have all but shattered the myth that being smart is not a part of the athlete's makeup. In fact, research shows that elite athletes are quite brilliant. Still, the dumb jock stereotype is yet another challenge for the gay athlete.

Today, the serious athlete knows that training smarter includes a certain amount of resistance training, and of course, that a certain amount depends on the discipline. Athletes today use the gym as an important cross-training tool, regardless of their sport. As a result, football and baseball players are finding themselves having to share the bench press and the dumbbells with the golfer, the swimmer, the cyclist, and the ballet dancer. Because of this, the athlete today not only fits into gym culture, he is an essential part and sizable faction within it. Raymond Pajek contemplates the roles that the gym plays in his life now:[3]

> [the gym plays] . . . a lot of roles. It is a place to exercise, and to enhance my athletics, because my primary interest over the last fifteen years has been on the athletic side, on the competitive side. But I also need regular stretching and strength training to compliment my workouts. Then it gives me something social to do. It's a nice place to see what other people are doing with their bodies. It's one of the few chances I get during the week to see people not fully clothed, with gym attire on, so I get a chance to admire people and also chat with people.

As far as gay gym culture goes, Scott remembers that:

> When I was coming out, one of the things I really wanted to do was meet other gay men who were like me . . . who were also athletes and into the outdoors. One reason I moved to San Francisco seven years ago was because I wanted to be in a larger gay community where I could be around other gay athletes, who were serious athletes or knew what it was like to have athletic goals and the commitment of training for something.[4]

Since antiquity, athletics and the gymnasium have been synonymous. Of course, sports happen outside the gym, but athletes use the gym to train and cross train for their sports as well as a place to socialize with and meet other athletes. For the athlete, the gym and the sport are more of a lifestyle than for the rest of us, often, the gym is, for the athlete, more than their *third space,* it is their *second home*. Today, the gay athlete holds a significant piece of the gay-gym-culture pie. But as Scott Robinson reminded us, the words *gay* and *athlete* have not always mixed well. Because there is not much in literature in terms of gay athletic history, it becomes important to question if the gay athlete is a new phenomenon or has simply come out of the closet.

A NEW PHENOMENON OR OUT OF THE CLOSET?

In ancient Greece, homosexuality and athletics went hand in hand. In modern times homosexuality and athletics have, for the most part, been mutually exclusive—so what is different? In much of this book I break down and examine stereotypes in an effort to understand them as well as their cultural influences. This method of deconstruction helps us understand the cultural constructions of a given group created and held by the popular mind. This method is particularly useful when it comes to both the homosexual male and the male athlete.

Both words of the phrase "gay athlete" are as new as the definition of the phrase itself. To fully understand why this is so, we must look at the two parts of the whole, the homosexual male and the male athlete, as separate entities that, until recently, have been mutually exclusive. This exclusion becomes a bit easier to understand when we examine the contradicting cultural constructions and definitions of each entity. As concepts and social entities, interestingly enough, and in terms of modern history, both "the male athlete," and the "homosexual male" are not only relatively new, they both entered the popular language and embodied stereotypes at around the same time.

The word "homosexual" was coined in 1869 by the writer Karl Maria Kertbeny in a pamphlet that he published anonymously in which he advocated the abolishment of Prussia's sodomy laws. In his groundbreaking pamphlet and subsequent writings Kertbeny argued that the criminalization of homosexuals violated the "rights of man." It was Kertbeny who, at the same time, also invented another interesting word: heterosexual.[5] Eleven years later, the term "homosexual" made it into academia when Gustav Jäeger, a professor of zoology and anthropology at the University of Stuttgart popularized the term in his book *Discovery of the Soul* (1880).[6] The word then gained recognition among the medical community when the psychiatrist Richard von Krafft-Ebing, who was in favor of homosexuality, published *Psychopathia Sexualis* (1886), which was a study on what was then considered deviant sexual practices (Krafft-Ebing's work was eventually the starting point in the medical practices of two better-known figures: Sigmund Freud and Carl Jung).[7] Soon thereafter, "homosexual" was made truly famous and entered the mainstream vocabulary via mass-media injection during the trials of Oscar Wilde in 1895. Although from the beginning "homosexual" meant same-sex sexuality, it was used mostly to describe male homosexuality and "homosexual" became representative of the male homosexual.

In 1896, the first modern Olympics were held in Greece. Only males competed in the first modern Olympics (events for women were added four years later at the Paris Olympics). Though the word "athlete" was not new, the practice had for the most part been dormant for almost 1,500 years. With the rebirth of the Olympics the "male athlete" became again a real person and not a conceptualized historical figure. As professionalism entered athletics, the athlete gained social status. Soon after, the professional athlete described the male athletic ideal. The birth of the modern Olympics in combination with the rise of a growing middle class in both Europe and America in the late nineteenth century resulted in sports gaining popularity and the male athlete quickly became the symbol of masculinity, youth, and virility. In a nutshell, the male athlete quickly became representative of the perfect specimen of modern man. Once again, as in ancient Greek times, the ideal man was modeled on the young athlete—or on the image of the virile, masculine, youthful athlete. As sports became professional, the professional male athlete achieved celebrity status and became the idol for both the young and the old, and for men and women. Even today, only the movie stars and rock stars rival the status that professional athletes hold in pop culture. The multimillion-dollar salaries and endorsements enjoyed by professional athletes are the best indication of how much the American public idolizes them. The onset of the modern Olympics was cause for both sports and the athlete to reclaim the status and respect they had once held during the Golden Age of Greece; only this time with much greater magnitude, as the modern Olympics were no longer limited to the inclusion of a few Greek states, but were now a worldwide event.

In direct contrast, the homosexual male was dealt a very different hand of cards—undesirable, despised, and persecuted, to name a few. Just as sports and the athlete were becoming all the rage, the trials of Oscar Wilde brought the topic of homosexuality to the mainstream media. For the first time in modern history "the love that dared not speak its name" was given one: Oscar Wilde. The male homosexual, in the public's eyes, was quickly modeled in the fashion of the famous Aristocratic Dandy. The stereotype attached to the male homosexual was defined as effeminate, weak, refined, and as the outcome of the trials would have it: immoral and illegal. In the minds of Victorian society, he represented exactly the opposite of what had become idealized and valued in men, he represented the opposite of the male ideal—the opposite of the male athlete.

In any case, both newly redefined concepts were in the minds of modern man, new as much as they were also mutually exclusive. Clearly, and only until recently, the phrase "male homosexual athlete" was considered an oxymoron. One word represented the idealized version of healthy and robust masculinity; the other, a newly defined pathology that threatened masculinity. Of course, as discussed in Chapter 2, this concept would have been ridiculous to the ancient Greeks whom had fashioned the ideal and for whom sex and relationships between men was not only a normal part of life, but a normal practice of male athletes.

As I discussed in Chapter 1, one cannot argue that a stereotype is an "oversimplified opinion," an "uncritical judgment."[8] Yet the stereotypes that have defined male athletes and male homosexuals are an incredible example of the power behind these oversimplified opinions. The defining characteristics of both stereotypes were opposites and in turn, to the popular mind, this is what created the illusion of an improbability. Not just in the world of sports, but in the world at large. While it is true that many male athletes are masculine and virile, so are many homosexual men. And while it's true that many homosexual men are effeminate, so are many heterosexual men. The conflict gets complicated because both stereotypes are right and they are also wrong. The male athlete and the homosexual male are people, sometimes the same person, sometimes not—sometimes masculine, sometimes not. The stereotypes associated with each, are just that, stereotypes—they are cultural constructions, not the reality of most men.

In decades following both the trials of Oscar Wilde and the onset of the modern Olympics, both stereotypes defined modern men and were unchallenged for almost a century. Then the 1970s happened, and the Sexual Revolution and the gay liberation movement came out in full force. Although it took some time, professional male athletes started coming out as well, challenging an even more robust stereotype: the assumed heterosexuality of the male athlete.

It is no surprise that for many gay men today, the idea of the gay athlete and the field of gay athletics are still, in their minds, somewhat of an anomaly. This situation is probably also one of the main reasons that gay cultural critics become uncomfortable with gay gym and body culture, as well as gay athletics, because they believe athletics, sports, and the gym to be antigay by nature. But the antigay sentiment in sports and athletics is a social construction, which has emerged from the meaning that has been attached to the long-held and inaccurate stereotypes of both the male athlete and the homosexual male. To attach ourselves to the notion that the gym or sports are antigay only helps to enforce and keep in place the erroneous stereotypes, not deconstruct them.

"I love sports like cycling and swimming, I'm a total athlete," a fellow cyclist tells me on a bike ride. "It's the ball sports I didn't like when I was growing up. When I was a kid, every time I turned around, someone was throwing a ball at me. It used to freak me out."[9]

An interesting phenomenon is that the *type* of sports rather than all sports become threatening to some gay men. Although the question could become an entire book on its own, it is worth asking: Why do the dynamics of contact sports make them threatening to some gay men like my cycling buddy? Invariably, it is the contact sports, those that involve a team (e.g., football, baseball, soccer), which seem threatening, rather than those that are less team-oriented where little or no contact between team members is encountered (e.g., swimming, running, cycling). Why the disparity? The most obvious answer is that in a contact sport team environment the social constructions and perceptions of stereotypes are enforced and there is more social pressure to be "like the other guys." Whereas in individual sports, you can train and compete on your own, and thereby be less subjected to social pressures, which results in the same social constructions and perceptions proving themselves wrong.

The power of stereotypes is tremendous. To get an idea of just how much, let's take a look at an institution where the social constructions of stereotypes thrive over reason.

HIGH SCHOOL ATHLETICS

> In high school I was erotically interested in other men, but a lot of it was a denial period for me, because I didn't really come out until I was twenty-four. Before that, I dated women and I felt like I was supposed to be part of this straight culture, and I kept trying to figure out how to make that fit with what was going on in my head. (Raymond Pajek)[10]

In few places are the powers of stereotypes stronger than in high school. Coming of age is a tough process of building identity, of searching for our place in the world. Leaving little room for close introspection, teenagers tend to explore and play out the identities of stereotypes that are already in place, especially those that are, in popular culture, ideal, such as movie stars, actors, and professional athletes—all of whom work hard to maintain the idol image granted them. The lack of gay role models and (out) gay ideals (movie stars, actors, and professional athletes), and the in-your-face heterosexuality of pop male icons give young gay men the impression that they are made of a different cloth, a process that not only results in social isolation but enforces all that is erroneous about stereotypes, both gay and straight. Today, the beliefs that all male athletes are heterosexual and all homosexual men are sissies are not just in your gay history books—they are drilled into the psyches of high school students every day.

For gay boys who are not athletic, the high school environment is often a very uninviting one; for those who are athletic, the same environment is tolerable as long as one's sexuality is concealed. The *jock* in high school is the ideal male teenager, the alpha male. Chances are that you have heard or read countless stories, coming from gay men, who felt isolated and excluded by not fitting in whatsoever with the stereotype. Gay boys who do fit the stereotype often stay closeted for years because there is a strong message attached to the stereotype that homosexuality does not fit the jock image. Fear of ridicule, among other potential dangers, drives even those who recognize their homosexuality to conceal it at all costs.

Raymond clearly remembers experiencing same-sex attraction in high school athletics:

> My first eye candy were fellow swimmers on the high school swim team. I specifically remember being fascinated with a few of the guys that were beyond having a boy's body, they had sort of already made that transition, they had abdominal muscles, and shoulders, they just looked more masculine than the rest of the boys did on the team.[11]

Yet, as much as Raymond might have enjoyed the "eye candy," being in the locker room and playing sports with other boys he was attracted to was also a fearful and conflicting situation:

> I had to conceal my attraction to them, or at least try to. Some gay men are good at being buddies with all the straight guys, but for me I was more inclined to just withdraw from the social activities that happened in the locker room. You get a group of straight boys together and there's a lot of socializing that happens in the locker room because they feel safe, they're away from girls, they're in a peer situation. For me it was always intimidating because I really felt that if I was going to play along acting straight, I was going to expose myself, because I knew inside that I was different, and I felt that the only way to protect that was to be silent. So when I was in locker rooms, I was always very quiet and tried to stay away from the fray. It was scary . . . very scary, because I was always afraid of being outed if I looked in the wrong direction or I gave some inclination that I was checking somebody out.

The homocentric nature of sports offers young men, gay or straight, a level of intimacy that is hard to find in other social arenas for men. For Scott, the camaraderie of sports offered an outlet for same-sex attraction as well as a time-consuming distraction from dealing with such:

> Athletics was an outlet for me up until I was twenty-nine, because I wasn't out. In a sense it was very erotic, to be training with another man. In some ways athletics satisfied the sexual urges—being in the locker room and taking a shower together. Before I was out it would give me an erotic charge.[12]

Given the conflicting environment of high school and youth athletics it is understandable why some gay social critics and many gay men become uncomfortable with gym culture—gay or straight gym culture. In high school, the gym and athletics were some of the most obvious places where gay boys did not fit in. Because the gym is associated with athletics and athletics are associated with homophobia, the conclusion is that the gym is homophobic. However, homophobia is a learned behavior. As I have stated previously, sports or the gym are not homophobic or anti-gay by nature, prejudiced people are.

Today's gay gym and gay athletic subcultures not only fight this homophobia, but are also slowly breaking down and redefining the stereotypes of the gay male and the male athlete. After gay liberation, a way to address the homophobia in sports was to organize gay athletes. As a result the term "gay athlete" is no longer an oxymoron; gay athletics are not just a reality but also a thriving success. The gay athlete is not a new phenomenon. Gay athletes have simply started coming out of the closet.

HISTORY OF MODERN GAY ATHLETICS

An interesting twist adds flavor to the history of modern gay athletics, one that is almost unknown and much less obvious. Before gay men were known as respected athletes they had gained notoriety as party boys. With the onset of gay liberation, much of gay life revolved around the bars and bathhouses in the cities that became the gay ghettoes. In short, gay life was one big drinking and sex party. Some things never change, and as it is now, moderation was often absent in the lives of many gay men during the 1970s. Alcoholism and drug abuse was rampant, and the depression associated with both led to an alarming number of deaths and suicides in cities like San Francisco and New York City. As a response to the problem, a few concerned community leaders and members came up with the idea to develop healthy social alternatives for gay men. One of those people was John De Cecco, who remembers the episode as part of his "political coming out."

De Cecco was a member of SIR (Society Individual Rights) in San Francisco and he remembers that in the early 1970s:

> SIR had been in operation only five or six years. It was the only gay rights organization for men in the city. They raised money through the bars. The parties would move from bar to bar, there were always more bars, more parties. Some of them began to realize there was a drinking problem. The mental health program started because the drinking got so bad that they were literally killing themselves . . .[13]

The mental health program De Cecco refers to was connected to Lavender U. Lavender U was basically an academic ensemble put together by community members (including De Cecco and other members of SIR) that organized around the gay movement and, in the form of a newsletter, started to offer and list courses pertaining to the self-enrichment and empowerment of gay men.

> The idea came from a couple of guys, Jack Baker and Gardner Pond, who were evidently joggers, to start the Lavender U Jogging Club. So we did, and we would meet on Sundays at different people's homes, and we would run along Sunset Boulevard, Golden Gate Park, and sometimes along the beach. There were only a small number of us who participated; I hadn't done anything like that in my life. I got as far as jogging around Lake Merced [4.5 miles] and started to realize not to take the body for granted. We would then have brunch afterward, and the brunches moved from home to home to home . . . and then of course the brunch included a lot of screwdrivers, and a lot of mimosas. The drinking never really disappeared.[14]

On their runs through Golden Gate Park the formidable group of visionaries was lucky enough to attract an unlikely coach. That coach was Tom Waddell, one of the most remarkable gay athletes of our lifetime. De Cecco, who knew Waddell on a first-name basis, told me that:

> Tom had been an Olympian, and he took an interest in what we were doing. He would get us running and he would give us advice on how to do it, how far to go, what to do with your food, and so on. He was our coach. So then the focus became very much the activity, the athletic part, and less about screwdrivers. I don't think Tom was much of a drinker at all, he had a kind of Puritan attitude about it.[15]

The academic part of Lavender U was later absorbed by what is now the Harvey Milk Institute in San Francisco, and the Lavender U jogging group changed its name to *Frontrunners* (named after Patricia Nell Warren's 1974 gay-themed and wildly successful novel, *The Front Runner*). Soon afterward, other gay running clubs formed around the United States and then later worldwide using the same name. The Frontrunners eventually incorporated into a full-fledged athletic organization, and today Frontrunners is the largest (and now oldest) gay athletic organization in the world with hundreds of chapters around the world and thousands of members.

Involvement in the gym and in athletics continues to serve as an antidote to alcohol and drug abuse and addiction. As a personal trainer, I have worked with several clients for whom fitness was yet another approach to staying healthy and focused, and away from self-destructing substances and behaviors. In my research, I found that 4 percent (224) of survey respondents listed "recovery" as one of the reasons they are involved with the gym and athletics (see Figure 6.2).

Social critics have often implied that gym culture has replaced the more "cultural" practices of old gay life, such as reading or attending the opera or the symphony. In my survey I also placed the question, "Did the gym or working out replace something in your life?" Although a few respondents did in fact say that they read less or were less active in cultural events, the majority of answers from the 17 percent (874) of respondents who said "yes" fell under two categories. One group said that the gym replaced "Boredom and being fat," "Eating, and being depressed," and "Sitting on my ass doing nothing."

The others said that the gym replaced, "Partying and drinking," "Drugs and clubs," "Being an alcoholic," and "Alcohol and smoking."

THE GAY GAMES

> Welcome to a dream that is now a reality . . . Welcome to a celebration of freedom.
>
> Dr. Tom Waddell, Founder of the Gay Games
> Kezar Stadium, San Francisco, August 28, 1982

Tom Waddell was one of those extraordinary men who were truly ahead of their time. Waddell played football and competed in track and field while attending Springfield College. After college, Waddell joined the army, but as a contentious objector refused to go to Vietnam. In turn, the army sent him to Fort Sam Houston where he trained as a decathlete for the Olympics. At the 1968 Olympics in Mexico City he placed sixth in the decathlon. Following his military career, Waddell attended medical school at Stanford and became a doctor specializing in infectious diseases.

Waddell had adopted San Francisco as his home just as the gay and lesbian liberation movement was beginning to flourish. It was there and then that he came up with an idea for the concept that has now turned into the worldwide famous Gay Games. It was a crazy idea for the 1970s, and one that would have probably not taken place anywhere else but in San Francisco. But after all, he was in the San Francisco of the 1970s. The first Gay Games happened there in the summer of 1982.

San Francisco Arts & Athletics (SFAA) was founded by Waddell in 1981, with the sole mission of producing the first Gay Olympic Games. Waddell's goal in the production of the Gay Games was to:

> Encourage athletic participation by gay men and lesbians, many of whom had felt marginalized from athletics . . . to promote the pride and self-respect of gay men and lesbians everywhere.[16]

The production of Waddell's Gay Olympic Games came to a halt when the United States Olympic Committee (USOC) obtained a temporary restraining order forbidding the SFAA from using the word

"Olympic." As a temporary response, the SFAA renamed the event "Gay Games" and in 1982 produced the first event at Kezar Stadium in San Francisco. One thousand three hundred fifty athletes showed up to compete in eleven sports, an additional 300 cultural participants joined in as well. For the second Gay Games, also in San Francisco, participation more than doubled in the number of competing athletes, to 3,500, the number of sports jumped to seventeen, and cultural participants to 400.

In June of 1987 The U.S. Supreme Court ruled against Waddell and in favor of the USOC, forbidding SFAA to use the word "Olympic." The following month, Tom Waddell died of AIDS. (The long-time legal battle, no doubt, contributed to Waddell's illness. He even had to sell his house in San Francisco to pay the fines that were ordered by the Supreme Court and the USOC; in the end he died a poor, beaten man.) After Waddell's death, The Federation of Gay Games was formed to take over SFAA and "perpetuate the Gay Games according to the founding principles."[17] Since then, the Federation has produced Gay Games III in Vancouver, IV in New York City, V in Amsterdam, The Netherlands, VI in Sydney, Australia, and VII in Chicago. The Federation recently elected Cologne (over Johannesburg and Paris) for Gay Games VIII, scheduled for 2010. A brochure promoting the 2002 Gay Games in Australia reads:

> Since 1982, Gay Games has been a powerful force for positive change around the world. Perpetuating and safeguarding the Gay Games and its founding principles of inclusion, participation and the pursuit of personal best is what the Federations of Gay Games is all about. Please join us.[18]

So far, Gay Games V in Amsterdam holds the record for most participants and sports; claiming 14,000 participants in thirty-two sports. Sydney follows them with 12,000 participants from seventy countries around the world competing in twenty-nine sports. (The long distance and costly expense of traveling to Sydney from the Western Hemisphere explains the decline in participants.) Gay Games VII were originally scheduled to take place in Montreal in 2006, however disagreement over logistics between Montreal and the Federation of Gay Games resulted in the Federation choosing Chicago instead and Gay Games VII took place there in 2006. The event drew 12,000 participants in thirty sports. In any case, Gay Games V, VI, and VII drew more athletes and participants than in the actual Olympics, an authoritative statement in sheer numbers alone, and an even more powerful message of presence to the rest of the world. The message of the Federation of Gay Games is clearly getting across.

Following the dispute between Montreal and the Federation of Gay Games, Montreal decided to host its own gay sporting event anyway. A new and rival event, the first "Out Games" took place in Montreal also in 2006. Out Games in Montreal drew another 12,000 participants (since the event took place only a week apart from the Gay Games in Chicago it appears that very few athletes attended both events and instead chose one over the other). While it's too soon to tell whether the Out Games are here to stay and gay athletes will have the choice of not one but two quadrennial larger-than-the-Olympics sporting competitions, one thing is for sure, gay athletics are now a tour-de-force.

It's a sad reality that great men often don't live long enough to witness the power of their dreams. Tom Waddell had many callings; he dared to be a serious dreamer, and one of those big dreams came true when the first Gay Games drew 1,350 athletes. The 14,000 queer athletes competing in Gay Games V in Amsterdam or the 12,000 who showed up in Sydney, or Chicago, or Montreal would have exceeded even Waddell's wildest dreams. Nevertheless, he left us a legacy, and Waddell's vision to promote the self-respect and pride of gay men and lesbians everywhere through athletics continues. Today, events like the Gay Games and Out Games are influencing gay men around the globe. Other venues around athletics continue to evolve for different causes from promoting athletics to raising money for AIDS. Of these other athletic events, in the last decade and a half, one of the most important cultural occurrences influencing gay athletics has been the AIDS Rides.

THE AIDS RIDES

The AIDS Rides were the brainchild of Dan Pallotta, another well-known jock. To raise funds for many communities ravaged by AIDS, in 1994 Pallotta originated the first California AIDS Ride, a seven-day, 560-mile, camping, bike ride/fund-raiser from San Francisco to Los Angeles. The first ride was a huge success and was recreated every year in California. Similar rides were staged in several other states, as far north as Alaska and as far south as Florida.

One of the leading factors in the success of the AIDS Rides is that the promoters seductively and aggressively recruited thousands of riders and volunteers. The riders and volunteers then created a word-of-mouth campaign, raising millions of dollars. After receiving an incredible amount of media attention, the AIDS Rides became a cultural phenomenon, and in the gay community, almost a trend. The rides became so popular that in California the ride would "close" to potential riders and volunteers several months before the actual event.

Eventually, the AIDS Rides became more than just about fundraising; they became a moving city of people with a powerful message, raising awareness and millions of dollars. As with most athletic events the environment could be considered cultlike. One of the most interesting aspects about the AIDS Rides was the variety of people in the riders and volunteers. The riders ranged in age from seventeen to well into their seventies; they came from every gender, race, ethnicity, socioeconomic status, and sexual orientation. It was a true melting pot of people.

Regardless of who you were or where you came from you still had to get on your bicycle and ride it for 560 miles in seven days—a serious athletic challenge. Yet the AIDS Ride promoters were not just recruiting athletes, but everyone else as well. In fact the majority of the riders who completed an AIDS Ride had not necessarily been athletic or done much serious cycling. They became athletes in training for the event. Because a large number of participants came from the gay community, the AIDS Rides were responsible for encouraging thousands of gay men who had never been athletic to pursue athletics. As a rider who completed three of the California AIDS Rides, and a trainer who trained several men and women to do the same, I can assure you that regardless of what shape you were in to start with, completing an AIDS Ride gives you the radical notion that you can complete almost any other athletic endurance event. Stories abound of many people who, after completing an AIDS Ride, went on to become serious and even competitive athletes.

The AIDS Rides were important not just because they promoted gay athletics in and outside the gay ghettos, but because through them the gay community was actively involved in educating the mainstream public not just about AIDS and HIV, but about queer people in general. Thousands of riders, a good majority of them gay, proved wrong the stereotype that gay men were not athletic. Another interesting factor of the rides was that they were part bike ride, part carnival. Many riders would ride in costume, sometimes in drag or makeup, etc. They were a gay tour-de-Mardi Gras. Masculinity was not necessarily part of the equation, and camp was often present. But at the same time, the ride represented a serious physical challenge; this didn't just challenge the stereotypes about gay men, masculinity, and athletes—in significant numbers it stared it right in the face—sometimes in full drag.

Because of their vast popularity throughout most of the 1990s and early 2000s, on a local and community-based level the AIDS Rides have been responsible for introducing cycling and athletics to many queer people in countless small towns and large cities across the nation. They were also one of those still rare events in modern day in which large numbers of both gay and straight people came together for any reason. While the Gay Games promoted athletics, it was geared mostly to gay men and lesbians who already considered themselves athletes. The AIDS Rides convinced the nonathlete that he or she could do something as athletically demanding as riding a bicycle from San Francisco to Los Angeles. Because of the large number of participants, the many millions of dollars raised, and the physical demand the rides required, the AIDS Rides were a bold statement of brute force reckoning with kindness. They roared *we've got muscle,* and a lot of it, and we're doing something really powerful, kind and important with it.

The fundraising logistics of the AIDS Rides spurred enough controversy to lead the rides and the company that produced them to their final collapse. In 2002, Pallotta Teamworks ceased operations and produced its last AIDS Rides. Since then, some of the organizations that directly benefited from the rides have begun to produce their own rides with limited success. It's too soon to tell what will become of the AIDS Rides; we have only the very recent past to analyze. But during the time that Pallotta was behind the scenes, on a cultural level, the rides were very successful in promoting gay athletics. Whether training for the next Gay Games, for one of the AIDS Rides, or for a local 10K or triathlon, gay men around the world are doing so in large numbers. By doing so, each and every one of them is slowly deconstructing the old stereotypes. Because of these stereotypes, and the demanding requirements of training, being a gay athlete can still be challenging in both our personal lives and when it comes to fitting into mainstream and even gay culture. Nevertheless, it has never been easier to be both a gay man and a male athlete. The scenario of acceptance however, takes a sharp turn into a dark tunnel when the gay athlete is a professional one.

PROFESSIONAL SPORTS AND THE ATHLETIC CLOSET

Since before the onset of gay liberation, gay men and lesbians in America have fought a long battle for acceptance and inclusion in the work force, with careers ranging from corporate America and politics to academia and blue-collar labor. In the arena of professional sports, however, we have unfortunately made a lot less progress, and when it comes to that American dream, the professional gay athlete has yet to take a bite from his piece of the pie. Although there is huge gap in the success and desirability level between male and female athletes, the gap between gay and straight athletes is even bigger. Nowhere is this gap more evident than in professional sports. This gap in acceptance and desirability is one of the most confining closets a gay man or lesbian could possibly experience: the *athletic closet* of professional sports.

As I have discussed, stereotypes are a very strong force in modern pop culture; in professional sports they are *everything*. Almost as defining now as they were 100 years ago, the concept that a gay man can fill the jockstrap is in the popular mind a very conflicting one.

A professional athlete must weigh a lot of factors when deciding to come out—factors that are deeply affected by the homophobia that is still such a part of pro sports. As Jim Buzinski, editor and CEO of Outsports.com told Mubarak Dahir of the *Advocate:* "Sports is one of the last great bastions of homophobia."[19] Fear of losing their jobs, their sometimes multimillion-dollar salaries and endorsements, and of being ostracized by their peers are the most common reasons as to why thousands of professional gay athletes are still in the closet.

In the 2,500 hundred years since the dawn of professional sports there have been gay professional athletes—from the Greek athletes, Dioclese and Sporos competing in the ancient Olympics to Tom Waddell and Greg Louganis contending in the modern ones. So it is a fallacy that professional athletes cannot be gay. Of course, to prove the fallacy wrong we need evidence, and this evidence comes in the form of professional athletes acknowledging their homosexuality. In modern times, more and more professional athletes have been courageous enough to come out publicly and begin breaking down the sturdy walls of the athletic closet.

Out Pro Athletes

One of the first gay athletes to come out was David Kopay, whose nine-year professional football career included playing running back for the San Francisco 49ers, the Detroit Lions, the Washington Redskins, the New Orleans Saints, and the Green Bay Packers. Kopay was the first American professional male athlete to publicly acknowledge his homosexuality. He did so in 1975, three years after retiring from pro football. He came out in an article he gave to the now defunct *Washington Star.* The coming-out story was so shocking that a year later, the contentious athlete published an autobiography, *The David Kopay Story: An Extraordinary Self-Revelation,* which became a *New York Times* best seller.[20]

Not long afterward, in 1982, Glenn Burke (1952-1995), a professional baseball outfielder for the Los Angeles Dodgers and Oakland Athletics, came out publicly as well. Burke, who is credited with inventing and popularizing the "high-five" greeting so commonly used in sports, had a much shorter career than Kopay. The span of his career was cut short, according to his autobiography and many other accounts, due to the homophobia he encountered by team managers. He died of AIDS in 1995.[21]

In major league baseball the two most prominent players to come out since Burke have been former umpire David Pallone in 1990, and Billy Bean in 1999. Pallone was fired from his baseball team in 1998 for allegedly being involved in a teenage sex ring (the charges were later considered baseless). Two years later the publication of his autobiography told a different story. In *Behind the Mask: My Double Life in Baseball,* he contended that the real reason he was fired was that he was gay.[22]

Nine years later, Billy Bean who had played (1987-1995) for the Detroit Tigers, Los Angeles Dodgers, and San Diego Padres came out in a front-page article in *The New York Times*. In the *Times* interview, Bean described hiding his homosexuality by staying married to a woman for nine years and even playing on the day that his lover died of AIDS. He has since become an avid spokesman for gay rights. His autobiography, *Going the Other Way: Lessons from a Life In and Out of Major League Baseball,* was published in 2003.[23]

As I am writing this book, you can easily count the handful of professional ball players who have come out. From active players in the NBA, the NFL, and major league baseball, what we *do* have is a long list of "I'm not gay" statements by numerous players and quite a few apologies for antigay remarks by both players and coaches. More interestingly, we do have a couple of "why I'm not coming out" stories that have been published. One of these is told by journalist Mike Freeman in his book *Bloody Sundays: Inside the Dazzling, Rough-and-Tumble World of the NFL,* in which he documents the story of a current football player with the NFL who is gay and closeted and who also claims that there is currently a "secret society of some 100 to 200 gay and bisexual NFL players"—a figure Freeman disputes.[24]

Two other professional football players have come out since Kopay, both of them after retiring from the sport. In 1992, Roy Simmons came out on the *Phil Donahue Show* and his story, *Out of Bounds: Coming out of Sexual Abuse, Addiction, and My Life of Lies in the NFL Closet,* was published in 2006.[25]

Most recently, the biggest name to come out from the closet of the NFL has been Esera Tuaolo in 2002. Again, his coming-out story sent shockwaves through the locker rooms of the NFL. The revelation came in the form of a front-page article in *The Advocate,* an article in *ESPN The Magazine,* and on television on *HBO Real Sports*. His announcement caused a controversial media frenzy that brought to the light the mixed bag of emotions that both his former teammates and other NFL players felt with the coming-out story. Tuaolo's autobiography, *Alone in the Trenches: My Life As a Gay Man in the NFL,* was published in 2006.[26]

Although the sentiments at the NFL vary spectacularly, a great number of fans have stated that they do not object to a professional player coming out. A poll taken by ESPN in 2002 found that when fans were asked the question: "If your favorite player announced he was gay, would that make a difference to you?" an outstanding 78 percent of respondents said "no," meanwhile only 22 percent said "yes." Levels of acceptance varied from state to state, with Hawaii ranking as high as 89 percent and Alabama and Mississippi as low as

52 percent; overall, however, in every single state the majority of respondents still seem to support a gay player coming out.[27]

In February of 2007 we had another interesting first when John Amaechi, a retired professional basketball player, became the first NBA player to come out. Amaechi came out on the television show *Outside the Lines* (ESPN) and ESPN books released his autobiography *Man in the Middle* the same month.[28] The gay-related dialogue in the locker rooms of the NBA has now begun.

Although most gay pro athletes are still afraid to come out, times have, and continue to change, and those who do come out effect change in the right direction. In America, there is a huge difference in possible outcomes between the times of Kopay and now. Although sports such as baseball, football, and basketball are the most challenging environment for a gay male athlete, other team and individual sports seem to offer gay athletes a little bit more tolerance and inclusion. Actually, take that back. Tolerance and inclusion was not offered, it was created and demanded by the few, brave—truly heroic—athletes who've come out in the midst of their career.

Outside of football, baseball, and basketball, in the United States and around the world, gay professional and Olympic athletes have publicly come out, while playing, in just about every sport ranging from snowboarding, rugby, and tennis, to skiing, swimming, and diving. An entire book could now be dedicated to summing up the coming-out stories of professional athletes that have taken place since David Kopay took that first step. Some of the most famous are former Mr. Universe Bob Paris and four-time Olympic gold-medal diver Greg Louganis, both of whom also published their memoirs. When it was published in 1977, Kopay's autobiography was alone on the shelf; today one shelf is not enough to house the autobiographies of gay professional athletes. Outsports.com, the leading gay sports Web site in America today, keeps a growing list of out gay athletes—a list so long that the question is not whether gay athletes exist, but rather why it is that some people stupidly believe that they do not.

In the athletic closet of ball-playing sports there is a bomb ticking: it is just a matter of time before one of these not-so-tough guys works his way up to having the *cojones* that many of his peers in other disciplines constantly exhibit. Of course, Mr. Professional Gay Ball Player will face many challenges, no doubt. But when he does and demands to keep his job and to be treated with the respect that he deserves, in the history of gay rights he will score a homerun, a touchdown, and a slam dunk all at once. And in doing so, he will not only write gay history, and become one of its true heroes, but also will significantly revolutionize the history and future of professional sports. This however is a very complex line of reasoning, after all we need to remember and respect the fact that these men set out to become ball players, not gay heroes.

Conclusion

The stereotypes of the gay male and of the male athlete have begun to change, but these changes take time to truly inject themselves into the mainstream. Every time you read anything about a professional gay athlete the words stereotype or cliché are always part of the thesis. The message is always the same: I am not the stereotypical gay man, I am a masculine ball-throwing jock, and I'm gay. The problem with a statement of that kind is that the same statement reaffirms the belief that there is a stereotypical way to be gay, and it is not athletic. Nevertheless, the statement even in its contradiction deconstructs and weakens the stereotypes. Gay gym culture in general is influential in reshaping this stereotype, whether the gym goers are athletes or not, because on many different levels, it disproves the stereotypes. This has begun to happen, and a new identity is reshaping the male athlete.

We now know that you do not have to be feminine to be gay or queer, that gay men are both masculine and feminine with every possible variation in between. At the Olympics, Gay Games, and the many sports events around the globe, gay men, lesbians, transgendered, bisexuals, questioning, and straight men and women participate in athletics. The "gay athlete" is no longer an oxymoron: gay athletes jump, play, catch, and kick ass as much as and sometimes better than heterosexual athletes. Gay athletes are as diverse as can be; they come in every color, shape, size, ethnicity and race.

With the increased popularity of gay athletics, gay men are reclaiming a field that they very much created: the athletic movement of ancient Greece. Queer people have proven to be brilliant in every field, from philosophy and education to mathematics and science. It is going to take time and a few more brave men and women to take the step and come out of the athletic closet. As they do, one by one, these men and women will, no doubt, change the world.

Chapter 9

The Circuit Boy

Corey Jennings

At the White Party in Miami, it was hard to keep my eyes from watching Corey Jennings (a pseudonym), a thirty-four-year-old from the Midwest, who was across the dance floor from me. At 6 feet 2 inches tall and 200 pounds of muscle shaped into the V-torso typical of underwear models, with six-pack abs, big chest, big shoulders, and seventeen-inch arms, Corey stood out from the crowd. His jeans were loose, and they dropped three inches below his belly button as he danced, displaying his ripped pubic area and in back the top two inches of a bubble butt worthy of its own calendar. When he got up on a box to dance, people watched and took pictures, and Corey loved every minute of it.

Corey, who is also a physician and an accomplished athlete, tells me that in terms of gay gym culture he identifies more as a circuit boy than anything else. There are two major factors that describe a circuit boy: a passionate affair with music and dancing, and the cluster of physical characteristics that are the circuit boy aesthetic. The circuit boy body is a gym-built body, often shaved in order to enhance muscular definition, but more significantly, the archetypical circuit boy is handsome and sometimes pretty. Their reputation is such that in gay culture, pretty or handsome muscle boys typically get classified as circuit boys, whether they are or not. One of the biggest myths about gay gym culture is that it is made up of circuit boys primarily. In this chapter, I address this myth and other associated myths about gym culture while also taking a look at the intriguing world of circuit boys. This chapter, while focused on circuit boys, is also about those who look like them.

Muscle Boys: Gay Gym Culture
Published by The Haworth Press, Taylor & Francis Group, 2008.
doi:10.1300/6034_09

THE CIRCUIT

> Since the beginning of recorded history the male members of the species have joined together in ritual dance. Adorned, semi-naked with rhythm instruments, they used this tribal rite to celebrate their gods and themselves.
>
> The Saint 1980-81 opening season membership invitation[1]

The "circuit" originated from a dichotomy: one, a celebration of gay life; the other, its most menacing threat.

Circuit culture was started by a group of well-off gay men who, given the freedom to openly socialize that gay liberation brought in the 1970s, would travel to places that would later become popular gay destinations. This jet set started meeting men from other cities, and soon they began designating weekends to meet at different destinations. A weekend in Miami's South Beach, another in California's Palm Springs, yet another one in New Orleans . . . eventually the itinerary became known as *the circuit*. The Saint in New York City's West Village and the Red Party in Columbus (both popular gay venues in the late 1970s and early 1980s and defunct now) are believed to have greatly influenced the trend as gay socialites jetted between the two venues on big holiday weekends.

For many gay men, the new gay lifestyle was one big party. Then the plague struck. In this, circuit parties also tell the history of gay culture and its courageous response to adversity. It is no coincidence that the rise of the circuit culture occurred in the early 1980s. The gay community was devastated: gay men—young and old, rich and poor, black and white—were turning up everywhere with the "gay cancer" (HIV had not yet been identified). Before long, the flourishing gay cultural centers of New York, San Francisco, and Los Angeles were fast becoming ghost towns. Money was desperately needed for research, treatment, and, once the virus was discovered, for prevention and education, yet the government's response was slow and minimal. For a long time, while thousands of gay men were getting infected, even then-president Ronald Reagan refused to acknowledge and even utter what he thought was a *gay* four-letter word: AIDS. Faced with death, members of the gay community came together like never before; many of them were the same men who traveled the circuit. Among many different types of fundraisers, they began organizing big theme parties to raise the needed funds: circuit parties.

As the 1980s progressed, the price of air travel fell, the disposable incomes of gay men rose, and the circuit gained popularity among middle-class gay men (urban, suburban, and rural) across the nation and around the globe. They take place in just about every major U.S. city and many of the smaller ones; they are also popping up in European and Latin American cities: Boston, Birmingham, and Barcelona to Paris, Prague and Puerto Vallarta. In the early 1990s there were just a few circuit parties in the United States, by the mid-1990s there were about fifty; there are now hundreds of circuit party events in cities across the world. As AIDS services became increasingly available, circuit events played a lesser role as fundraisers. Party promoters stepped in, capitalizing on the phenomenon. Now, while many of the events still provide funds to charity, many others are for-profit venues.

A circuit party usually refers to a weekend rather than a single event. It's a collection of parties, typically over long weekends, which culminate in one major extravaganza party. Thousands of people attend each circuit party: gay men, mostly, but a few straight guys, and some women, both straight and lesbian.

One of the biggest and most popular circuit parties in the United States is the White Party held in Miami every fall, typically over Thanksgiving weekend. I attended the twentieth annual White Party in 2003 with a group of friends, and while the goal was to party, there were so many parties that we attended only one of the events each day. The schedule of events for the weekend and information about them took up four full pages in *Wire,* a popular weekly in Miami's South Beach (SOBE).

Circuit party weekends typically start on Wednesday and end on Monday. The "Women's" events are predominantly geared to lesbians; the straight girls, for the most part, hang out with the circuit boys.[2]

Here's an example of a circuit-party agenda from *Wire.*

Wednesday

"White Knights VIP Reception," (7 p.m.-10 p.m.): Cocktail pool party, $50.

"Victory Party," (11 p.m.-5 a.m.): "Official after party of the White Knight's event," $15.

Sin Leather (9 p.m.-3 a.m.): Leather and fetish dance party, $10/$15.

Thursday

"White Dining," (noon-8 p.m.): Thanksgiving dinner party, $20.
"White Starz," (10 p.m.-5 a.m.): Dance Party, $20.

Friday

"Heat Wave Pool Party," (noon-Sunset): Cocktail pool party, $15.
"White Party Shopping Event," (7 p.m.-9 p.m.): Cocktail fundraiser/party, free.
"White Dreams," (9 p.m.-6 a.m.): Dance party, $85/$95.

Saturday

"White Noize—Unbound Afterhours," (5 a.m.-1 a.m.): After hours dance party, $15/$20.
"Muscle Beach Party," (noon-sunset): Beach dance party, $30.
"Cirque Blanc," (9 p.m.-3 a.m.): Women's dance party, $25/$30.
"White Heat," (9 p.m.-5 a.m.): Dance party, $50.

Sunday

"Wet Tea Dance," (noon-6 p.m.): Women's cocktail pool party, $10.
"White Dawn," (8 a.m.-3 p.m.): Morning dance party, $25.
"White Party at Vizcaya," (6:30 p.m.-11:30 p.m.): The official White Party, $150.
"Noche Blanca @ Crobar," (10 p.m.-5 a.m.): Dance party, $75/$85.
"Noche Blanca @ Space 34," (10 p.m.-6 a.m.): Dance party, $45.

Monday

"White Horizon," (6 a.m.-5 p.m.): After hours dance party, $30.
"Relax," (10 p.m.-5 a.m.): Dance "official closing party," $20.
"Swan Song," (7 p.m.-5 a.m.): Party hosted by local gay bar, no cover.

At most of the events, prices include admission only; drinks will run anywhere from $5 to $10. Most of the dance parties take place at large (okay, huge) nightclubs, some as big as 16,000 square feet. The Annual White Party at Vizcaya is held at the magnificent Vizcaya Museum & Gardens. The pool parties are held at trendy and upscale SOBE hotels (like the Delano Hotel, where supermodels and movie stars are known to spend their weekends).

Music is the soul of the circuit. The most expensive events are the most popular and most attended, and, as a rule, they offer the hottest disc jockeys (DJs) in the gay world: Tracy Young, Victor Calderone, Susan Morabito, Manny Lehman, and Tony Moran, all of whom are celebrities within the circuit set and sometimes outside of it. (Tracy Young, for example, has been known to DJ the private parties of music celebrities such as Madonna, Lenny Kravits, Ricky Martin, Lauryn Hill, and Sean "Puffy" Combs.) This explains, at least in part, the hike in admission prices, as celebrity DJs earn anywhere from $5,000 to $20,000 per event, sometimes more. In addition, the biggest parties will sometimes also present a live performance, if not several, by MTV-famous pop stars as well as cameo appearances by other music, television, and movie celebrities.

So many parties, so little time. But most important, so many circuit boys—thousands and thousands of them in fact—which brings us to the beefiest part of the circuit.

THE CIRCUIT BOY

John Putnam is a thirty-two-year-old paramedic who lives in Los Angeles. Just before moving to Los Angeles in 1998, his best friend back in New Orleans, where he was born and raised, introduced him to circuit parties, and that year he went to two different circuit events, which were enough to captivate him:

> It is a culture that I never knew existed. I realized that there are thousands and thousands of gay men out there who are masculine, they have great bodies, they're normal guys. It's nice to look around and see masculine guys, and that makes me feel good about myself and to know that I'm a part of this group.[3]

Thirteen percent of my survey respondents identified with circuit culture (see Figure 6.1), although many others noted that they occasionally attend a circuit party or two but not frequent enough to feel that the circuit makes up a big part of their lifestyles.

Circuit culture mirrors the party boy subculture of urban America, and is largely made up of urban muscle boys. As John points out, the masculine aesthetic prevalent of muscle boys is also part of the circuit boy aesthetic. Although the majority are young, white, and middle class, circuit culture includes every age, socioeconomic class, color, and race. The ages and socioeconomic status of circuit partygoers range anywhere from college students and twenty-somethings, who work just to pay their way to circuit party weekends, to white-collar professionals in their thirties, forties, and fifties.

Regardless of the many demographic differences that make up circuit culture today, there is one common denominator found in circuit boys, and that is the gym-built body. Like Corey Jennings and John Putnam, circuit boys across the country and around the world spend a considerable amount of time at the gym. Most circuit events, like the White Party in Miami, include beach or pool parties in which no more than shorts or a swimsuit make up the dress code. In addition, eveningwear is basically pecs and abs as shirts and tank tops are either coat-checked or left to hang from low-waisted jeans—the majority of partygoers go shirtless once they walk in the door. Because there's so much skin at circuit parties, the chiseled muscular build has become the nucleus of circuit culture. So much is the muscled body a part of circuit culture that today many in the gay community routinely refer to a built and muscular body type as a *circuit boy body.* This association begins to explain why the circuit boy aesthetic and gym culture have become interchangeable.

Although most people wish to be in better shape, after attending a circuit party for the first time, as one circuit boy states, the desire "multiplies tenfold. You see these big, buff, beautiful guys and you want to get bigger and more muscular." From the fliers used to promote the parties, to circuit magazines and Web sites, the message that a hard lean body is a must is more than obvious. More so than any other subgroup within gay culture, a hard and muscular body is the most valuable trait at any circuit event. One of the major realities of the circuit party scene is that you'd have to be crazy to hang out at circuit parties and not work out. Basically, if you are going to party on the circuit, you are going to hit the gym—a lot.

CIRCUIT TRAINING

> I want to know that whenever my favorite song comes on I can rip my shirt off and feel good . . . I don't want to hide; I don't want to cover up anything. So do I work out for the good of circuit parties? No, but circuit parties certainly do remind you that you gotta go to the gym.[4]

If you were to spend an entire day at a popular gay gym in New York City, San Francisco, Los Angeles, or Miami, you could observe that besides circuit boys, there are only two other male subgroups that give their workouts such priority and importance: athletes and professional models. I have, on many occasions, noticed circuit boys who spend more time at the gym than athletes who are preparing for competition. It is not unlikely for circuit boys who work out on a daily basis to start going to the gym twice a day during the two to three weeks before a circuit event. This type of dedication and the physical work involved does indeed turn the circuit boy into an athlete, albeit a *cosmetic athlete.* From an exercise physiology standpoint a great number of circuit boys are not just fit for athletic competition but sometimes in better shape than competitive athletes (in fact many circuit boys eventually develop a serious interest in athletics and pursue athletics on both recreational and competitive levels). In any case, because many circuit boys approach their training—*circuit training*—with the diligence and dedication of athletes and supermodels, they reap the same physical benefits and when it comes to the circuit, the desired outcome: the body beautiful.

> Of course you can go and dance and have a great time and not have the greatest body. It's not forced, it's not a weight that the circuit scene puts on people. People choose to go into the circuit scene . . . and that's part of it, it's having a great body, so either that's your scene or it's not, and if you choose to go into that scene and you like to work out and be healthy then it makes sense.[5]

Circuit parties are often talked about (and just as often criticized) because they are recognized as assemblies of beautiful men. But beauty as a whole on the circuit is defined more by the appearance of the body than the traditional definition of beauty based on the face.

What has really occurred within the circuit and in much of pop culture today in defining male beauty is a wider definition; it now includes the broadening and definition of the major muscle groups on the male body. Beauty is then defined less by classic or traditional beauty, as we know it, and more by the body beautiful.

Although the definition of beauty is still limited, this is progress, because beauty then becomes a more attainable ideal. More important it is an ideal based on the healthy and empowering practice of physical fitness. This is the ideal around which circuit culture thrives. After all, it is much more realistic and healthy to build a beautiful body than a beautiful face. More than anything, it is the body beautiful that creates all those "beautiful men," because what *is* indisputable is that the majority of circuit partygoers are in above-average shape.

The high premium that the body beautiful assumes on the circuit is grounds for some circuit boys to do everything they can to get as big and muscular as possible. Besides countless hours at the gym and as many dedicated to nutrition, a number of circuit boys will, just like some athletes, get *juiced*.

In the 1990s, Scott Cullens was one of Los Angeles's top personal trainers. Scott was co-owner of L.A. Health Management, a group of personal training studios in Los Angeles and New York City that catered to Hollywood stars and affluent New Yorkers. With a client list that included actor Brad Pitt and supermodel Rachel Hunter, Scott and his gyms were a sensation and were written about in *Vogue, W, Allure,* and *Fitness*. The 1990s was his decade in the fitness limelight; it was also his decade to shine on the circuit. After going to his first White Party in Palm Springs, Scott remembers, "I jumped right in; once I started I didn't stop."[6] Scott then spent much of the 1990s well integrated in the then-rising circuit culture. He hit just about every circuit party there was to go to at the time. He also spent that time bodybuilding and using steroids to become one of the biggest boys hitting the parties. At 5-foot-10 and 185 pounds Scott was already naturally big and muscular. But when he was going to the circuit, bodybuilding, and on steroids, Scott was topping the scales at about 220 pounds.

Aside from training celebrities Scott also spent quite a bit of time training himself, often seven days a week. During his years on the circuit Scott Cullens experimented with several anabolic steroids, including Deca-Durabolin (nandrolone decanoate), testosterone cypionate, human growth hormone, Durabolin (nandrolone phenylpropionate), Anadur (nandrolone hexyloxyphenylpropionate), and Winstrol (stanozolol), to name a few. His steroid cycles were carefully planned and scheduled around circuit parties. "My cycle was timed so that it would hit at its peak when I hit the city limits of whatever city I entered. I had this down pretty good." Competition bodybuilders routinely employ this timing technique. The way Scott puts it, "You knew when you were going to look your best, and what you needed to get there."[7]

Anabolic steroids make circuit training more complicated. Many circuit boys are experienced bodybuilders who use the drugs responsibly and focus on risk reduction. What is problematic is that many who are not experienced in bodybuilding or well versed in anabolics also want to partake. I was talking to a popular circuit boy at the gym who has been working out only a couple of years and whose knowledge of bodybuilding is very limited. He told me he was going to start taking an anabolic steroid in pill form that a friend was going to get for him—and he could not even pronounce its name. In any case, anabolic steroids bring to the dance floors the complexities I have already discussed, from the potential for abuse and illegitimacy of the drugs to the legal risks of dealing with a controlled substance.

One common myth is that all muscle boys who use steroids are by default circuit boys. While sometimes true, most often it is not. Here we run into an interesting double standard. A lot of muscle boys have no problem obtaining the substances illegally and injecting themselves with the magic juice, yet look down at the circuit because of its association to *other* types of illegal drugs—those that they consider unhealthy. At other times, even when completely absent from judgmental attitudes, many muscle boys simply have no interest in the circuit for a number of different reasons. Nevertheless, I think it would be safe to say that in gay gym culture circuit boys as a group fall second to the poz jock in the consumption of anabolic steroids. However, because some circuit boys are also HIV positive, it is hard to tell who gets them prescribed and who does not, and almost impossible to define the line between aesthetics and survival.

Another myth when it comes to circuit boys is that they are all victims of body dysmorphia or what is also referred as the "Adonis complex." Body dysmorphia is a psychological, distorted body image disorder in which the person affected (mostly males) feels that he is not muscular enough even when he is built to bodybuilder proportions (it is often referred to as a type of reverse anorexia nervosa). Some circuit boys do suffer this condition, but I am convinced that most do not. Although the condition is complicated, a common trait is the amount of energy that people who suffer from it will put into covering up their body. The thought of putting their naked body on display is simply frightening to them. On the other hand, 99 percent of circuit boys often spend their entire weekends half-naked in front of thousands. In addition, body dysmorphic disorder is often diagnosed by how much the gym activities keep those affected from interpersonal relationships. For circuit boys, the gym activities are not only the basis for socialization, but working out is something they often do together. Many circuit boys spend two or three hours at the gym to complete a workout because they spend half, if not more, of that time socializing. Sure, circuit training is intense and time consuming, but that does not make it pathological. The elements of the circuit and the classical traits of dysmorphia simply do not add up.

The focus on appearance customary of the circuit is nothing out of the ordinary: in modern society a certain amount of grooming and a particular aesthetic is standard and expected for the corporate world, the academic world, and the athletic world; to suggest that the same should not be expected *and* accepted of the social-party world is unreasonable.

Whether built naturally, like John, or chemically enhanced, like Scott, there is no question that circuit culture motivates thousands and thousands of men to build themselves into modern-day Apollos. The interesting question then becomes why the circuit generates this kind of motivation.

We can begin to find the answer if we look into the essence of circuit boys: the nature of men. Through millennia man has never been able to divorce beauty from its evaluation. This process yields competition.

THE MR. CIRCUIT BOY COMPETITION

> Why do I dance on the box? I dance on the box to get noticed. I want to be noticed as much as possible, and I want people to take photos of me and talk to me. I don't just want to be one of the people in the crowd. When people see you and they take

your photographs and they want to meet you and they want to talk to you it's a big ego stroke.

Corey Jennings (pseudonym)[8]

The circuit boy trains like the athlete or the model because like an athletic contest or an audition for male models, the circuit party becomes a sort of competition, an unofficial beauty pageant. While other subcultures such as the leather and bear communities have formal and large-scale organized competitions (and many smaller ones) every year to elect the hottest leather man (International Mr. Leather) or the hottest bear (International Mr. Bear), the circuit party does not have an official competition—because the competition is built into the party. The circuit party is the contest; it is the fashion show; it is the unofficial Mr. Circuit Boy Competition. Simply put, it is the competition that drives circuit boys to take up the training schedules of athletes and underwear models.

We encounter competition in just about everything we do, from sibling rivalry when we were children to the competition we face at work and in the dating pool as adults. From the playground to the bedroom, and in many other facets, life itself is a competition. Unless you are living in seclusion, it is impossible to live a life without experiencing it. A certain level of competition is considered healthy, and the better we understand it and learn to deal with it, the better we can respond to it when it arises. Competition also encourages us to do better than we would otherwise, whether at the gym, school, or at work. In mating and dating, competition happens on many levels, and varies whether the goal is a long-term relationship or a single-serving one.

When Corey and I discuss how competitive he feels in training for and attending circuit parties, he tells me, "Subconsciously, I think a lot. I want to be the person about whom people say, 'Wow, look at him.'"

The more circuit boys I interviewed and surveyed and the more I thought about some of my friends and acquaintances who are also circuit boys I came to an important realization. Circuit culture attracts gay men who by nature thrive on competition, not just within the circuit, but outside of it as well. In Pscychology-101 terms, circuit boys as a group exhibit the classic type-A personality: a strong desire for recognition and the willingness to work and compete for it. Take Corey: besides doing what it takes to get through medical school, and besides hitting a few circuit parties a year, he also does triathlons *for fun*. Three years ago he spent an interesting day in Kona, Hawaii, starting with a 2.4-mile rough water ocean swim before getting on his bicycle for a 112-mile ride and ending the day by running a marathon (26.2 miles)—all in the name of completing that King Kong of athletic competitions, the Ironman Triathlon. Or take Scott Cullens: what kind of personality do you think it takes to go to Los Angeles practically unknown and become one of its top personal trainers, start a fitness business, and sell it a few years later at a tremendous profit?

In sports as in life, a certain amount of competition is considered healthy, but to what extent is competition healthy in the circuit?

> You can make it healthy. For example I think it's healthy when I feel that I look pretty good and work out to see if I can fine-tune a little bit, like getting my abs a little tighter. Then I'm happy. If I can get my chest a little bit fuller, then I'm happier. Unhealthy is when I'm doing what I just did: I just finished a cycle of steroids to get bigger, to get the bigger chest, to get the bigger arms, to get the tighter abs.[9]

Corey has done three cycles of steroids in the past two years and in the process he's gone from 170 pounds to 200 (when he did the Ironman he had not yet used steroids). No stranger to medicine and the risks involved, he makes sure to tell his physician when he's on a cycle and undergoes routine blood tests to "check my liver function, check everything that is going on with my circulatory system, to check everything." According to Corey, at least on the surface, circuit parties are his number-one reason for using steroids, but:

> I've always been thin. I will always see myself as thin; it's just my self-image, and this is a way to overcome that, by getting bigger. It all comes back to self-image and self-confidence, because people treat me differently now than when I was 30 pounds lighter. Even my patients do.[10]

Corey makes an interesting point: people *do* treat you differently when you pack on thirty pounds of muscle, whether you do it naturally or with the help of steroids. Muscular size, for the most part, commands attention, admiration and respect—in and outside of gay culture, and in and outside the circuit. This reality, of course, complicates the dialogue of working out to get bigger and even that of using steroids, because it is how external factors influence personal actions. Why steroids are popular on the circuit, where it's all about the body, is a no-brainer.

When I ask Scott Cullens about the relationship between his bodybuilding and the competition at circuit parties, he tells me that "I enjoyed it, I was building something, maybe nothing that was going to save the world . . . but it was a project that was kind of fun to me." But then he tells me, "I mean there's no sense of competing if you're not going to win."[10]

Competitiveness is of the essence when it comes to circuit culture. As Corey points out, you can make it healthy or not. Of course not everyone is competitive and because of this the circuit can be challenging and uncomfortable to the many people who instead thrive in less competitive environments (the type-B personalities). In addition, circuit culture is based on aesthetics, and when we combine this foundation with the reality of genetics, unfortunately not everyone can compete, even if they wanted to. Yet, how comfortable or uncomfortable someone might feel about the circuit quite often has nothing to do with personality types or genetics. The circuit celebrates not just the body but interpersonal relationships and sexuality in ways different from the outside world.

SEX, LOVE, AND THE GAY FRATERNITY

> Circuit parties are like family reunions with my friends . . . through the circuit parties I've met some of my best friends. One bad thing about meeting good friends through circuit parties is that they are all over the country. The number one reason I go to circuit parties is to get together with my friends; number two is the dance music. The t-dance, happy, bouncy, uplifting lyrics . . . is absolute ecstasy to me . . . to get away from work, away from the real world, away from any judgments from straight society. You're just out there on the dance floor, surrounded by your friends, surrounded by thousands of people that are just like you. To me there is no more free feeling in the world. I honestly feed off of those tiny little memories from month to month to month. I can be at work stressing my balls off and think about some anthem that I heard two months ago and stop for a second and smile.[11]

Unlike the athlete or the model, the circuit boy does not compete for a medal or a photo shoot, but for something closer to the heart: potential mates, both platonic and romantic. Often the two are connected, but before we talk sex and romance let's take a look at the platonic aspects of the circuit.

The desirable outcome when it comes to competition is a sense of recognition. In circuit culture such recognition comes in the sense of inclusion. Many circuit boys such as John and Corey report experiencing a sense of brotherhood; because of this, circuit culture mirrors the dynamics of fraternities. Building a circuit boy body is the ticket to joining the fraternity, and the socialization among like-minded gay men is the foundation that holds the circuit together.

When Corey's not traveling to circuit parties, which he does about five weekends a year, his life back home is about as unlike that of a go-go boy as possible. He is a successful physician in private practice. "Day to day I deal with an older population, a very conservative population, and it gets boring and mundane," he tells me.[12] For Corey, circuit parties are a great antidote to dull work; they also present the opportunity to meet like-minded gay men:

> You get to be around other gay men who work hard at the gym. At the circuit parties I get to see a lot of people I met at other parties—it's the only time I see them again, so it's a way to stay connected with people. It's a way to get out, to blow off a lot of steam, and just to have a lot of fun.

One of the least explored yet most worthwhile effects that circuit culture has on gay society is the camaraderie that many circuit boys report. This is important, especially for gay men, because many of them have never felt included. In addition, it gives us perspective into that complex realm that is the self-esteem of gay men in general and not just circuit boys.

Most people who have watched Corey dance shirtless and smile when other men ask for his picture would not even entertain the question, "Do you feel you have low self-esteem?" The answer came immediately as his tone of voice and his eyes dimmed from vibrant to sad: "Yes," he said. The young hot doctor—who owns a beautiful condo in the best part of town, who drives an expensive car, and who also happens to have a charming personality, great looks, and a body that could give any porn star a run for his money—also has a past that includes a childhood familiar to many gay men:

> I never fought in high school, and I used to get picked on. I was very thin, and I was smart, I was in music, even though coming from a very small school I also played sports. But I got picked on, I got picked on by kids six years younger than me . . . the *scarring,* a lot of it comes from when you're very young versus when you're older.

When we dig a little deeper, we often find that that the circuit boy story is really *our story.* My experiences in talking to so many circuit boys have convinced me that the circuit attracts many gay men who are trying to heal old wounds. A lot of circuit boys embrace (or try to embrace) the lifestyle in order to overcome past shortcomings in social interaction. Given the homophobic environments that plague most gay men's childhoods and adolescence, it is no surprise that many feel a need to make up for lost time, or at the very least, a place to fit in. This conflict is a well-known common denominator in most coming-out stories. It is exactly the essence of this concept: of finding fraternity at circuit parties, of feeling like they belong.

Many circuit boys develop close-knit friendships and groups of friends through the circuit scene and find significant outlets of social support and camaraderie. In addition, a number of both short- and long-term romantic and sexual relationships and experiences evolve from the social events.

Love and Sex

The *methods* we use to become more attractive are really less relevant than *why* we are willing to go to such lengths. I believe the answer can be found in those other irrational fascinations that drive men to even more unexplainable actions: *love* and *sex*. In our minds, the muscle studs at circuit parties inspire us to want and become one of them because we want to mate with them. Folk wisdom has taught us that whether we want to love them or just bed them, if we want to get with them, then we must become like them. The most beautiful are almost always the most sought after. I am convinced that at circuit parties, where the competition is fierce, what drives us is more Darwin's survival of the fittest than Freud's narcissism.

Circuit parties are the place where circuit boys compete for romantic partners. An endless number of romantic partnerships evolve from the events; many couples on the circuit have met their partners at one of the events. Some of these relationships flourish into long-term commitments sometimes spanning years and even decades, others last just the weekend. One of the interesting dynamics about the circuit when it comes to relationship models is that it does not really have one. Within the circuit you can find classic and monogamous, marriage-like relationships—lots and lots of them. But you also find that many others are anything but traditional and anything but monogamous.

Aside from the scheduled parties, at any circuit party weekend are an endless number of private cocktail parties, sex parties, and orgies. Sex is a huge part of the circuit party appeal. Like most good gossip, much of the hype surrounding circuit parties really boils down to sex. If we take a closer look at the type of fun that goes on at the weekend-long parties we would come up with an interesting list: half-naked boys dancing the night away, sex parties, orgies, nonmonogamy, and overt celebration of the flesh—all behaviors, acts, and attitudes that violate the unwritten code of ethics of modern queer culture that basically aspires to mirror the failed model of heterosexual marriage. Cultural critics have bashed circuit culture because like bacchanals of ancient times, there is a paganlike element to circuit parties in which sexuality, and the body are openly celebrated and accepted. These facts alone are enough to make our Judeo-Christian-Puritanical society very, very uncomfortable.

Yet, whether we like it or not, it is exactly these unapologetic pagan-like attitudes in regard to sexuality that have made the circuit wildly successful. The rise and success of the circuit is solid proof that for a huge number of gay men, predominant societal standards of normalcy and decency are not just completely irrelevant but for many, completely hypocritical. Although many conform to such norms back home, they also go to great lengths to escape them. The reality, (and a lot of people don't like this), is that many men—both gay and straight, and within the circuit and outside of it—are often much more interested in getting in touch with their *inner stud* than pursuing the classic heterosexual-monogamous types of relationships. It is male biology, that's all.

Because there is so much sex at circuit events, unsafe sex (barebacking), and the transmitting of sexually transmitted diseases, these events have become a problem for circuit boys and an arsenal for cultural critics. In response, organizers and health community organizations consistently get involved to promote safe-sex measures and education at most of the events. The prevalence of barebacking and sexually transmitted diseases in gay culture are a serious problem, true, but they are not specific to the circuit, as the problem is prevalent wherever gay culture thrives. It is a bigger problem of the gay community.

PARTY DRUGS

Just as at any other large-scale nightlife celebration, "party drugs" are part of the equation. Party drugs are both part of the appeal as well as a challenge when navigating the circuit. The most popular drugs at circuit parties are Ecstasy, GHB (gamma-hydroxy butyrate), and methamphetamines, all known to induce euphoria and provide the user with incredible amounts of energy. The most common reasons that circuit boys give for using the drugs are to enhance the circuit party sensory experiences relating to the music, lights, touch, and sex. In addition, the party drugs provide circuit boys with the energy for the party and sexual marathons that take place at circuit events. Less explored and less acknowledged is the fact that party drugs also play an incredible role when it comes to dealing with the issues of fitting in, competition, body image, and sexual taboos—both inside and outside the circuit.

Some circuit party attendees don't use street drugs, or if they do, they do so responsibly. At the White Party in Miami I met a thirty-year-old Florida native who goes to three or four circuit parties a year and he does no drugs at all. He told me that:

> I've tried a few of the party drugs when I was younger and just didn't really enjoy them. I especially didn't enjoy the hangover afterward. I don't even like to drink for the same reason. When I go to a circuit party I go there to dance and have fun and can do both without any drugs or alcohol, and I have a blast.[13]

Of course, when the topic is drug consumption we come up against some serious challenges: the potential for abuse, overdoses, and other mishaps. When I ask John Putnam, the Los Angeles paramedic, which drug-associated problems he sees most frequently, he answers:

> Mainly at circuit parties, the biggest one is GHB (which is a sedative-hypnotic, often compared to a liquid form of ecstasy). The other things are minor in comparison to that; hardly anyone drinks alcohol at a circuit party so that's not even an issue. Mainly it's GHB overdoses—I would say that's 90 percent of our patients.[14]

The rest of the problems, John said, come from overheating or drinking too much water after taking Ecstasy. Although many circuit boys take ketamine or "Special K," he rarely sees an overdose. Crystal methamphetamine users tend not to crash and find themselves in an ambulance: "Crystal doesn't take you out," John says, "it keeps you going."

How much of a problem drugs are on the circuit is directly proportional to the individual characteristics of those who use them. In discussing an entire group of people, it is very difficult, if not impossible, to pinpoint when and where and for whom the drugs become problematic. But from my observations and research, I think that on the circuit, the bell-curve model could very well apply. That is, we find a small number of people who do not use the party drugs; a large number of people who use them but for whom the recreational drug use does not become problematic; and last, a small number of people who use the drugs, often abuse them, and develop serious drug-related problems.

Although sometimes drugs are a problem, many people are addressing it. For one, a great deal of circuit events (and all of the major ones, I believe) now come with a team of medical volunteers like John who are there specifically to deal with drug mishaps, potential overdoses, dehydration, and any medical emergencies. In addition, as Corey told me, "It's a problem, but I think more and more people have seen somebody get into trouble with them, so in the back of their head people are watching each other or realize it and try to slow down a bit."[15] Other organizations present on the circuit, such as Party Safe (partysafe.org), focus on promoting risk reduction.

Another interesting point that needs to be made—and one that critics of the circuit ignore altogether—is that at gay events one will typically encounter a lot less mayhem, drug-related or not, than at straight events, whether it is a sports event or a Saturday night circuit party.

Having bartended at popular nightclubs in California and Florida that hosted both straight raves and gay circuit parties, I have experienced and observed this phenomena first hand. At one large nightclub with a capacity of over 1,000 partygoers in Florida, where I spent a few months bartending, and which hosted both gay and straight events, the number of security guards or "bouncers" jumped from one or two on a gay night to ten on a straight night! Even though the security staff was made up of all straight males, each of them preferred to work the gay nights over the straight ones simply because security problems, especially fights, were almost nonexistent on those nights. Is it possible that more chaos occurs on a Saturday night at your local straight nightclub than over an entire circuit party weekend? Absolutely.

In today's gay world many of us go through phases of partying and sometimes being reckless—it comes with being young. Scott Cullens no longer is interested in circuit parties or in bodybuilding. He recently moved to Palm Springs with his partner of two years, and the two are starting a new business venture.

> I couldn't go back to that place or ever want to be that person again, but that person made me a better person now. The experience was extremely valuable. I have a healthier relationship with my soul and with my body.[16]

GUILTY PLEASURES

From the Greek festivals of Dionysus before Christ, to the Roman bacchanals after him, people have spent considerable amounts of energy, time, and money on the precious pastime of having fun. Modern American life and the responsibilities that come with it leave so little time for fun and playtime, that those who make the time for it often get socially penalized for it. Our European counterparts who are used to two- and three-month vacations shake their head in disbelief when we tell them that the typical annual American vacation time is two weeks. In America the association between pleasure and guilt is so pervasive that we actually use the phrase *guilty pleasure* to describe those things and actions that give us satisfaction and enjoyment and are not work-related. Whether ordering the creme brulé for dessert or taking time out to read a thriller or romance novel, we have come to accept guilt as part of the equation. Scott Cullens remembers the time he spent on the circuit as "more fun than should have been allowed by law, well actually *was* allowed by law in most states . . . I feel pretty lucky being able to look back and think I had so much fun!"[17]

In many ways the circuit is a rite of passage for the young gay men who partake, a phase that they go through while exploring self-image, friendships, and sexuality. After all, the beauty of the boys and lifestyle of the circuit are both by nature impermanent; circuit boys don't stay young forever. Although some men go to five or six circuit parties a year, others go to a circuit party once a year and others even less. And while there are circuit boys who make a career of the circuit, most men who hit a circuit party now and then have a complete life outside the circuit, and like Corey, John, and Scott, are important and valuable members of our society.

The body often becomes too much the focus of circuit events, and this of course can have its repercussions. However, there is another side to that coin, as we know ignoring the body is not healthy either. We cannot possibly disregard the health benefits of a *mostly* healthy lifestyle and those that come with building strong lean bodies. Taking care of our bodies, however, is a lifelong concern. Because the gym is an extension of the circuit party, it often becomes a healthy social outlet not only between circuit parties but even when the parties are no longer a part of a circuit boy's life. As we get older and health matters more and aesthetics less, this is critical in terms of the well-being of the community. There are challenges, no doubt, in developing a healthy and vibrant body image. Finding that healthy medium is crucial. Once we understand how we each deal with competition and how we can address the challenges in modern gay socialization, the same events offer the opportunity for men to explore their body image and sexuality while developing a healthy relationship to both mind and body.

In conclusion, the circuit offers the opportunity for young gay men to develop important social skills, build significant relationships, explore their sexuality and self-image, and take with them into the future the lessons learned. Of course, like in other areas of our lives and within any other subculture, all of these self and socialization factors pose challenges—those challenges we call Life.

Chapter 10

The Muscle Bear

Luke Cottrill

Standing 6-foot-3 and weighing in at 250 pounds, Luke Cottrill is one of the biggest men at the gym. Most people, he tells me, find it hard to believe he is gay, because he's so "not the stereotype." His colossal size—he's extremely muscular as well as fat—can appear intimidating to most guys on the street or at the gym. But Luke is not just big; he is usually the strongest guy at the gym—any gym. He can squat 450 pounds, bench press 350, and dead lift 500. Luke says that he does not "work out for symmetry and beauty; I train for strength."

Luke Cottrill is also a gay athlete—a world champion with a few gold medals under his weight belt. Cottrill is a competitive power lifter; he is what we have known throughout the ages as a strongman. In gay and gym culture today, people describe the medal-winning athlete as a muscle bear.

Luke is a stereotypical strongman in that he is big and burly, masculine, muscular, and super strong. Unlike the bodybuilder, the strongman is not defined by symmetry and conventional beauty but by mass and strength. As I discussed in Chapter 1, the ancient Greek ideal emerged from the strongman ideal. In Chapter 3, I further discussed how it was also a strongman—Eugen Sandow—who was responsible for founding the genre of bodybuilding. Whether we are discussing ancient gym culture or Victorian gym culture, strongmen have always played a defining role in the evolution and emergence of gym and body culture.

Strongmen have always been around; the real phenomenon today is the emergence of a group of homosexual strongmen and the subculture they have built around those physical traits that distinguishes them from the rest of us. Having adopted a new catchy and less pre-

Muscle Boys: Gay Gym Culture
Published by The Haworth Press, Taylor & Francis Group, 2008.
doi:10.1300/6034_10

tentious name, strongmen are now emerging as an influential group of gay gym culture—we refer to them as *muscle bears*. The typical muscle bear is beefy, and often overweight, but he differs from stereotypical bears in that he is also muscular—extremely muscular, sometimes. Muscle bears are also hairy and sport a blue-collar image and style, even though many, like Luke, are white-collar professionals and well educated.

In this chapter I will discuss the formation and emergence of bear culture in the past two decades, then I will describe how the muscle bear became a new phenomenon in bear culture, and how these muscle-enhanced bears are becoming an influential segment of gay and gym culture. Finally, I will discuss the paradox of a group of men who once renounced the body and are now increasingly defining themselves by it.

BEAR CULTURE

Gary Phoenix (a pseudonym) is a forty-nine-year-old architect who lives in San Francisco and identifies with bear culture. At least one of the reasons Gary identifies with bear culture is the way he looks, he stands 5 foot 8 inches tall and weighs about 180 pounds, he also sports a beard:

> When you go to the gay newsstand, and you see publications like *Out Magazine* . . . I look at that magazine and say there's nothing about me in here, I don't relate to any of this stuff.[1]

I met Gary at the gym, where you can find him two or three times a week, and for him the main reason for working out is "health, mostly health, and staying limber . . . Working out has kept my body from aging, it gives me something healthy to incorporate into my life, and it's improved my body image."

Bear culture surfaced in the 1980s in San Francisco, and in two decades has evolved into a full-fledged and rapidly growing worldwide community. Complete with bear art and bear bars, bears now have their own version of the gay flag, several books on bears and their admirers, a vast collection of bear porn, countless Web sites dedicated to bear admiration and community, a bear cruise and spiritual retreat, bear cookbooks, and even a short feature film about bear love:

A Bear's Story. In addition, a series of colossal bear-centered social events are bringing together bears from every corner of the country and from around the globe.

Gary, who is a veteran of bear culture, remembers at least in part why the movement started in the first place:

> I think bear culture started out as a reaction to the mainstream gay culture. It said, OK, we don't identify with gay culture, we'll reinvent gay culture, we reinvent by instead of incorporating what the media says we are, we'll make it up out of scratch and it'll be less stereotyped, less made up, more natural.

A bear will be the first to tell you that it is hard to explain how beardom became an international social movement. But everyone agrees that the bear movement originated in San Francisco in the 1980s, and because I lived in San Francisco during most of the 1980s and 1990s, I can offer a series of possible factors. Here is a straightforward picture of what was happening then in the city and its beloved and notorious Castro District:

Bear Factor #1: AIDS

During the early 1980s, AIDS ravaged San Francisco's gay community. Once vibrant and sunny, Castro Street became depressed and gloomy. Everyone was dropping dead. Fear was in the air. Hope was nowhere. In the disheartened environment that was gay San Francisco in the early 1980s, it is not hard to understand how a large number of survivors would not be influenced much, if at all, with the superficialities of beauty, aesthetics, and fashion.

One of the most notorious physical effects of AIDS was wasting. Wasting caused robust men to be reduced in appearance and vigor to a silhouette of the men they once were. Because of this, visually and metaphorically, to be big and even fat symbolized exactly the opposite of wasting and its deadly effects. In this sense we can compare bear culture to the many tribal subcultures throughout history that have idealized bigness and fatness because these traits were indicative of abundance and thereby survival.

In addition, the menace of the disease represented losing all strength and along with it that trait instinctive to how men put up a fight: their masculinity. Gay men at the time were unarmed and powerless. It is in the nature of men to feel emasculated when facing a total lack of power. And if nothing else, AIDS robs its victims of their power.

To some extent, bears and the poz jock are dichotomies of the AIDS epidemic. For bears, the threat that AIDS represents to the body and to masculinity can begin to explain how those who felt threatened would psychologically attach themselves to images and traits indicative of strength and masculinity. In a nutshell, to be strong and masculine like the ancient strongman became an understandable ideal. Strength and masculinity had never before symbolized so much for modern gay men; in the 1980s strength and masculinity correlated with staying alive.

Bear Factor #2: The Anti-Circuit

Bear culture is the counterculture to circuit culture. The two cultures clash. The suggestion that bear culture evolved largely out of an anti-circuit sentiment gets thrown around quite a bit, but it is usually blown out of proportion. That bear culture has come to represent an anti-circuit ideal and that it has become an alternative to the circuit is true. In the 1980s bear culture was as new as the circuit. The circuit party and its body ideals were propagating, true, but this was happening in other places, like Miami and Palm Springs, not in San Francisco's backyard.

Besides, the circuit revolves around conventional beauty ideals, and while San Francisco is known for many things, an abundance of beautiful men is not one of them. As a young gay man who was visiting from New York recently told me, "the men here are not really good looking; there are no pretty boys." While not entirely true, such a statement is fairly accurate if we compare San Francisco with New York, Los Angeles, or Miami. If a lack of people who can fit into an ideal is not present, then that ideal cannot flourish; in San Francisco, traditional beauty ideals or people fitting these ideals are not the standard. San Franciscans, gay and straight, are better known for being laid-back scruffy intellectuals who are indifferent to conventional glamour—it is actually something we take pride in. In many ways, this is the perfect environment in which something like bear culture can flourish.

In any case, the circuit party was not a San Francisco gay ghetto incident. The circuit party was largely a phenomenon of another place and the next generation. It is a myth that circuit and bear culture have been or are mutually exclusive of each other. As I will explain later, it is more of an urban myth than reality. However, because circuit culture was an influential portion of gay culture, especially in gay media, during the same time that the bear movement flourished, it is quite possible that the circuits' prominence fueled the rise of beardom.

Bear Factor #3: Fashion or Antifashion Statement?

Bearness is largely based on a look—call it antifashion, or call it bear fashion. Although San Francisco cannot take credit for the circuit party, the city was the headquarters of even bigger fashion and social trends. Cornerstone of the Hippie movement and sexual revolution in the 1960s, San Francisco also saw more than its share of disco balls in the 1970s, and last but not least, the Castro was birthplace to the now legendary gay clone of the same decade.

From a fashion standpoint, the 1960s and 1970s were revolutionary. However, the 1980s has gone down in fashion history as one of its worst decades. Having been a teenager in the 1980s, I can tell you that when it came to fashion, well, as much as I hate to admit this, we were experimenting with some of the newest, not to mention most frightening, ideas the fashion world had ever witnessed: punk rock, mod, and new wave to name a few. (I will never forget the look of shock and fear on my mother's face, poor thing, when she came home from a vacation in Costa Rica to find my bedroom painted in black and me in it blasting *Culture Club* while sporting a new jet-blue Mohawk. That was my *mod* phase; it also was just the beginning of the decade.)

Many of the founding bears had been teenagers during the Hippie era of the 1960s and young adults during the Disco era. Having been fashion victims to bell-bottoms, tie-dye, platform shoes, and pompadours, who could blame these guys for renouncing fashion and pop culture? Really, you have to draw the line somewhere, and for young bears, the 1980s was the perfect place to do it.

Bear Factor #4: An Aging Community

Bear culture came about when the 1970s were over and the gay clones who survived the AIDS epidemic were arriving at middle age. Take a clone, add ten years, some whiskers and twenty pounds, and you've got yourself a bear. In this sense bearness can be explained as what happens to a lot of men when they get older.

So common is the bear look among middle-aged straight men that one has to wonder if bearness is more a result of middle age for males in general and less of a gay social trend. Prior to gay liberation there were no influential role models or precedents, there was no general consensus of what out gay midlife was supposed to be like; at least when one was somewhat masculine and out of the closet. If bear culture is any indication, maybe, just maybe, bearness *is* the model for gay midlife.

The mainstream media is only now discovering bear culture. In the spring of 2003, journalist Paul Flynn of the *United Kingdom Guardian* asked the million-dollar bear question in an articled titled: "Is the potbelly the new gay ideal?"[2] A few months later, having found a new identity (and a date to go along with it), writer Andrew Sullivan wrote another entertaining article declaring, "I am Bear, hear me roar!"[3]

People might draw different possible conclusions, but in San Francisco in the 1980s, all of these scenarios were happening simultaneously. Most likely, in one way or another, they all shaped and influenced the birth and evolution of bear culture. But regardless of how bear culture got here, it has now become the honey-flavored choice for more and more gay men. A great number of the constituency is middle aged, yet as the popularity of the hirsute grows, more and more younger gay men are giving it a bear hug.

Although it's difficult for bears to agree on exactly how the culture was started, they all agree that beardom is inclusive and loving of large body types and that at the center of their code of conduct is a post-gay celebration of raw masculinity. At least in part, one of the most obvious and interesting expressions of bear culture is its goal as an antidote to the conventional, sculpted, and hairless, underwear-model male.

BEARNESS

Nineteen percent (924) of the men who took my survey identified as a bear, and 28 percent (1,365) of total survey respondents identified as muscle bears. Many respondents identified with both of the categories, "Bear," and "Muscle Bear," but many of them only with one or the other (see Figure 6.1).

How does a bear become a bear? Well, for one, you have to look the part. Bear culture was founded on the principles of promoting acceptance of large and sometimes overweight body types. In the process, bears renounced mainstream manicuring of the male image: they enjoy one another's natural smells and facial and body hair.

Because bear culture's defining years occurred in the age of the Internet, bearness is no longer just a San Francisco social movement—it has become a national and international trend. In the United States, bear clubs and organizations have emerged in just about every city, big and small—and the same goes for a rapidly growing number of cities in the European Union.

In the United States, one of the largest and most prominent bear events is the International Bear Rendezvous (IBR), which is held every year in the bear motherland, San Francisco.

At the Ninth Annual International Bear Rendezvous 2003 in San Francisco, bears from around the world congregated for a jolly weekend of food, fur, and fondling. Hosted at the Ramada Hotel in downtown San Francisco, the event drew an estimated 1,000 bears.[4] The weekend included, among other activities, a teddy bear factory tour, a South of Market bar crawl, a Saturday night dance party, a beer bust, a Sunday brunch followed by a play (sex) party at a local sex club, and the pinnacle of the weekend: the International Mr. Bear Competition 2003.

The Mr. Bear Competition has become so well known worldwide that the same year contestants came from as far away as Perth, Anchorage, Knoxville, and Cologne to compete. Bear culture has become such a recognizable subculture of San Francisco that at the Mr. Bear Competition event, Assemblyman Mark Leno presented IBR organizers with a proclamation citing creativity and good nature and thanking them for their sales tax dollars. Another city politician, Tom Ammiano, also presented the IBR with a proclamation declaring February 16, 2003, International Bear Rendezvous day in San Francisco.

Looking the Part

Bears have defined themselves because of the way they look. This of course is somewhat contradictory—given that the founding principles of bear culture are based somewhat on the rejection of the body—the defining characteristics of bears are, for the most part, physical ones. Although some bears will argue that being a bear is not a look, it is a "state of mind," there is no denying that looking and acting the part is a part of the bear equation

Body Type

Bears are big guys who not only accept their large and burly figure—they worship it. The most defining and distinguishing feature of bears is their body type: they are mesomorphs and endomorphs. Bears are built like the animal they have chosen to adopt as their mascot and whose name they have taken: heavy and husky. Traditionally, the social dynamics of bears have revolved around eating and drinking. And it shows. Bears are accentuated by beer bellies and quite often, high percentages of body fat. If we use current medical definitions of body composition, bears are, in general, over-fat, and many are obese.

To their defense, however, the "over-fatness" of bears is questionable. In the fitness industry we are now learning that fit and fat are not mutually exclusive and that it is quite possible to be heavy and fit at the same time. Although this is an area of study still lacking sound scientific research, the concept is gaining momentum and acceptance. It is quite possible that the findings could result in new values of body fat for men.

Besides better health and aesthetic appeal, Luke Cottrill remembers other benefits to being a strongman:

> My friend Bob got sick with AIDS, and he was wasting away . . . and I was there to take care of him. And the nurses would come have to get three or four of them to move him . . . and I would reach down and I'd pick him up and he'd smile and say, "Nobody else can do this, Luke. See, that's why God made you big and strong, Luke, so you could pick me up.[5]

As difficult as the situation might have been, Luke was able to take a further step toward loving his body.

> It would be killing me, but I sense the truth to what he said. When I did that with him, that God always has a purpose . . . The bottom line is that on a good day, I can pick up the back of a car. Am I a universal type? No, I'm not a universal type, but that's OK . . . I like my body; I like my body a lot, and it's healthy and strong.

Hair

The second and most notable bear trademark is defined by fur: beards, mustaches, and lots of body hair. Although in much of gay—and now straight—culture, the standard is to wax and shave the male body, when it comes to body hair, bears just do not go bare. Quite the contrary: body and facial hair are celebrated. Some bears trim and shape their body and facial hair, others simply concur that the hairier the better.

So highly prized is facial hair in bear culture that many bears have not really seen their faces *without* hair in decades. Some bears I've talked to confess that they grew their beards and mustaches back in the 1960s and 1970s—mainly because it was the fashionable thing to do. Many of them simply haven't shaved since. This of course supports my theory that the shaggy bear look has been dramatically styled by the fashion and social trends that preceded it. After all, founding bears had survived, and were the product of a time in which the best-selling musical on Broadway was *Hair.*

Many people today are under the wrong impression that the smooth male is a new trend. Body shaving in males dates back 3,000 years to ancient Egypt and Greece. Back then, men, like now, shaved their bodies primarily for two reasons: to appear younger and to accentuate muscular definition. However, these are two particular traits unimportant and even undesirable in bear culture. So much is body hair a defining feature of bear culture that the lack of it is considered undesirable, and more specifically, not manly. This brings us to another defining and important characteristic of bears: masculinity.

Masculinity

Another sturdy and, according to bears, one of the most desirable and defining features of bear culture is a sort of raw masculinity. Their masculinity is displayed to a great extent by physical characteristics and appearance, especially the facial and body hair and the strongmanlike body. Luke, who is very butch and masculine, looks so tough that he was hired to model as a prison inmate in an ad intended to scare kids away from drugs. So much is a hard and rough appearance valuable to bears that bear culture has adopted blue-collar work wear as its clothing of choice, further accentuating a masculine and rugged look and in the process idealizing blue-collared men.

Because of this, from a cultural standpoint, one of the most noticeable dynamics of bear culture is the different socioeconomic classes of the group. Go to any bear event and you will find a diverse crowd of lawyers, bankers, and architects socializing with auto mechanics, bus drivers, and park rangers. This dynamic, which is hard to find among most other modern gay groups, probably has to do with the limited size of the group and can be compared to the founding gay culture of the 1970s, an environment in which homosexuality in itself was the common denominator. "I love masculine men," says Luke. "Ever since I was a little kid . . . I think it's something we're born with. We idealize femininity; we idealize youth; what's wrong with idealizing masculinity? I think masculinity makes you a man. As masculine gay men we need to reclaim our masculinity . . . it's OK to be masculine."[6]

The masculinity exhibited by bears is, as far as many bears and their admirers are concerned, their most attractive attribute. The motto of the now-defunct *Bear Magazine* stated "Masculinity . . . without all the trappings."[7] Such a statement of course sounds attractive to bears and nonbears alike who value masculinity. Unfortunately, when it comes to beardom, its most attractive feature also becomes it most significant—and less talked about—downfall. As Gary Phoenix told me:

> In the beginning, Bear culture was trying to invent a new way to look at masculinity and I thought that was very good, but it has instead embraced a lot of the lousy parts of masculinity, all of the guy-ness, insensitive crass.[8]

The social implications of such a high premium placed on masculinity results in a number of problems. For one, masculinity in bear culture is increasingly not just desired—it is required. We assume that men who look like lumberjacks and auto mechanics are manly. Folk wisdom suggests that being a big hairy guy is synonymous with being masculine. But to what extent is this true?

Although masculinity is one of the most desirable bear traits, the truth is that while for some bears it is an innate behavior, for others it is a performance—an illusion. For obvious reasons, this presents a serious problem. In order to define itself, the group is using not just outdated, but often unrealistic definitions of manhood. For men who have all the physical traits of bears and would like to be part of the group, but lack the masculinity, bear culture becomes downright bigoted. Still, some wannabe bears will butch it up and act the part. The irony is that for a culture that prides itself on avoiding drama, its prejudiced stand on masculinity puts many of its members through quite a bit of acting.

Attend a bear social event and you will notice that, like the rest of gay men, though many of these manly men *appear* masculine, they are *not*. Talk to enough bears and you will find out that while some bears are truck-driving, rough and rugged lumberjacks who live in the country, others are BMW-convertible-driving city slickers who work as interior decorators and live in lavish, pastel-colored Victorians. The truth is that the majority of bears fall somewhere between omega and alpha males. Once we make this connection, the bear community is very similar to the leather one: Largely made up of people who share a fetish or lifestyle that is practiced mostly on the weekends—white collar by day, blue collar by night. Though they might appear and dress like a lumberman for social occasions, this type of *metro bear,* from day to day is truly a bearded yuppie.

Bear culture, no doubt, was successful in reinventing a subculture of its own; however, the group's dynamics eventually devolved into the same type of insularity that they were rebelling against. As Gary told me:

> It came to a point when it got sort of overwhelmed by its own made-up culture. I think it became co-modified and marketed, and a whole world by itself that it has its own rules; instead of breaking the rules it invented new rules. I think it is still pretty accepting—one of the things that's nice about it is you go into a bar and there's people of all ages—but it's also become a formula. It's about dressing a certain way; it's about acting a certain way. I sort of imagined when it was born that it would integrate better into the rest of the world but it's become very, very insulate.[9]

Masculinity . . . without all the trappings? Negative—it's masculinity with the usual trappings.

Bear culture is clearly gaining momentum, and the new kid on the block is starting to get his share of the gay pie. In the process, it is creating change in gay culture and redefining long-held modern standards and ideals. But bear culture itself is changing as we speak. One of the most dramatic changes evolving out of the past few years and currently overhauling bear culture is a dramatic change in shape—literally, of bears themselves. As bears have begun hitting the gym a new bear has emerged. We are now witnessing a new ideal, which is quickly becoming central to bear culture, while at the same time redefining what it means to be a bear: *the muscle bear.*

THE MUSCLE BEAR

Jay DeMarco (a pseudonym) is a self-employed professional in San Francisco. The forty-six-year-old works out four to five times a week. The time he spends at the gym is obvious: at 5 foot 6 and 200 pounds he is massive for his height. His shoulders are wide, his chest bulges, and his arms and legs are muscular and thick. Jay has been working out since he was seventeen, and although he appears like a bodybuilder he doesn't identify as one. "The only reason I don't call it bodybuilding is because I don't compete, so I just call it lifting weights." Jay sports a goatee and plenty of body hair. He identifies as a muscle bear.[10]

Bear culture is quite new to Jay: "Three years ago, four years ago I didn't know what Bears were." Yet, much of his social life now revolves around bear culture—he hangs out with other muscle bears and they go to bear-centered parties, social events, and weekend getaways.

How the muscle bear got built is a process. The 1990s saw a huge, national emphasis on the promotion of health and exercise by both the medical and political establishments. Everyone was being encouraged to exercise, and the advice, this time around, was not coming from a suntanned, pretty boy with big pecs and a six-pack; it was coming from the Surgeon General and primary care physicians. People started taking the advice seriously. Exercise had arrived and it was receiving the mainstream recognition it had been seeking since the time of the ancient Greeks.

Some bears became concerned with their health and wanted to be in better shape. Others simply wanted to lose weight for aesthetic reasons. At the same time there was a rise in HIV infections among gay men, and the use of anabolic steroids in HIV management was becoming more popular. Anabolic prescriptions usually come with directions from the doctor to join a gym and start working out.

For reasons that range from the most genuine health concerns to downright vanity, in the late 1980s and early 1990s the gay gyms of the Castro, Chelsea, and West Hollywood started seeing an influx of bears as new members. What resulted was simple exercise science: regular weight and aerobic training will result in the building of the muscles and the loss of body fat. Bears got buff and blossomed into muscle bears.

Luke tells us:

> I think that people can be athletic and healthy and not be the stereotypical look. I think it's possible for a guy to be thin and healthy and sexy; I think it's possible for a guy to be musclebound and be sexy; and I think it's possible for a guy to be overweight and sexy. I'm one of those guys who are overweight, I'm never going to be thin, but I'm sexy. I go out and people hit on me all the time.[11]

Already a masculine icon, the muscle bear is not your regular bear—he is a gym-enhanced bear. Like Luke and Chris, muscle bears look like other bears with the exception that their bodies are much more muscular and have a lot less fat. Some muscle bears are naturally built with a sturdy muscular frame; most others, however, got buff and got leaner by going to the gym and lifting weights. Whether he got his strongman physique by genetics or by free weights, we know one thing: given the newly acquired object-of-desire status of Mr. Muscle Bear, it's working quite well for him.

When it comes to body image, muscle bears aim for bulk rather than definition. The biggest difference between a muscle bear and a typical bodybuilder is basically the percentage of body fat and the amount of body hair. In bodybuilding, low percentages of body fat and little body hair enhance muscular definition. In contrast, the muscle bear is not concerned with definition. Muscular bulk—fat and hair included—is the desired outcome.

Paradoxically, in the antibody-conscious bear culture, muscle bears became the new and improved version of the traditional bear. He appeared more muscular and more masculine and, as irony would have it, more desirable.

How desirable, you ask? Well, I asked the same question.

I interviewed a friend of mine who dabbles in bear culture. Across the gym is a tall, handsome, bearded, and very buff hairy bodybuilder.

My friend points him out and tells me that the man is one of the best-known bear porn stars who goes by the porn name "Jack Radcliffe." To put in perspective the star status of Mr. Radcliffe, my friend also told me: "He's the Marilyn Monroe of bear culture, he is the Leonardo Di Caprio of bears."[12] Mr. Radcliffe declined an interview for this book; he said that he did not identify with bear culture or with being an icon for that matter. However, a few weeks later at the Hairrison Street Fair (a new bear street fair in San Francisco) I watched as bears of all ages gaggled over the bear porn star like teenage girls over Leonardo Di Caprio. Contradictory to its founding principles, there are porn stars and starlets in bear culture.

To put it briefly, the muscle bear is the antihero of bear culture; he became the starlet, the porn star, and the sex idol for bears. He is muscular and buff—yet not ripped or interested in a lean midsection or a six-pack. Unless of course, it's a six-pack of beer, what better way to work on that sexy muscle-bear beer gut after all? He has average to high percentages of body fat, yet he is healthy and strong. He is involved in fitness and healthy lifestyles, but not overly concerned with being fit.

When it comes to body ideals, unlike the Falcon porn star, one of the strengths of the muscle bear as an ideal in gay culture is that it is one which is quite attainable by a greater number of men without considerable time investment. But not all men.

> The muscle bear thing is not something everybody can attain. It's something to strive for, as long as it makes you happy and you don't become obsessed with it. . . . There's this thing about our culture—the obsession to be perfect. And that is impossible.[13]

The muscle bear has quickly become the sex symbol of bear. Our strongman Luke has been asked to be in porn more than once. Although Luke has declined the offers, the fact that he is being pursued as a commercial object of desire is an indication that the standard definition of the body beautiful is changing and that there is increasingly a greater demand for alternatives. Yet the muscle bear is not completely divorced from the body beautiful: instead, body beautiful ideals have managed to infiltrate antibody-beautiful bear culture. The muscle bear is middle ground between conventional and unconventional beauty ideals and norms. This observable fact, porn stars aside, is best witnessed at most large-scale bear social events.

At the International Mr. Bear Competition 2003, the crowd of several hundred bears favored the buffest and most muscular of all the contestants, a sexy muscle bear contestant from Cologne, Germany. Mr. Germany was given the loudest and wildest rounds of applause and later that evening was declared International Mr. Bear 2003.

IBR is topped in attendance only by the now-infamous Lazy Bear Weekend held annually in sleepy Guerneville/Russian River, California (about two hours north of San Francisco). Although some bears would be mortified at the comparison, Lazy Bear Weekend has all the makings of a circuit party: pool parties, cocktail parties, dinner parties, afternoon parties, evening parties, late-night parties, even a slippery foam party at a nightclub. Lazy Bear is a social scene, drawing thousands of gay men from around the country and around the world, and revolving around big parties, where sex is quite central to the weekend and the buffest and biggest men become the event's superstars. Although many bears (especially the elders of the community) are not happy about this, as we have learned from Jay and Luke, more and more, bear culture is adopting social dynamics similar to those of the circuit. A bear circuit party is a circuit party. Lazy Bear has been wildly successful, and similar large-scale productions and weekend events, such as Bear Pride in Chicago, Phurfest in Phoenix, and Spring Thaw in Seattle, are also gaining popularity.

The embracing of bear culture by a younger population is sure to dramatically change the dynamics of the group. It is already causing a number of disagreements between the younger and older members of the group. At the center of these disagreements is the role of the muscled body typical of muscle bears and how this is antagonizing the founding ideals of the subculture. Another major disagreement, as I will discuss shortly, revolves around the use of party drugs at bear social events.

Whereas ten or twenty years ago bears were the social antidote to circuit boys, today the muscle bear can be defined as a cross between the circuit boy and the bear. When I asked Jay how he became a muscle bear, his answer was as honest as it was explicit:

> I was going to a lot of circuit parties, and I started looking at the guys that were bigger. I started getting more interested in them, so I wanted to get bigger. When I started partying (on the circuit) I was twenty-five pounds lighter. Honestly, this is what hap-

> pened: I did a lot of steroids and a little bit of human growth hormone, and I got much bigger and I grew more hair.[14]

For Jay, the transformation was a good thing because he had always been attracted to the bigger, older, and hairier guys; now they were noticing him—and he liked that. As he told me, it did not take very long for the circuit boy to ease into bear culture, "Next thing I know . . . presto! Change-o! I'm a muscle bear."

As Oscar Wilde told us, "The pure and simple truth is rarely pure and never simple." It turns out that sometimes the muscle bear is a hybrid created out of the past twenty years of gay culture. In fact, at the International Mr. Bear competition, I did not see many of the muscle bears that I know or recognize from the gym. When I asked some of them why they had not attended the event, many of them said they were actually a few blocks away, partying with the circuit boys at a monthly circuit party called Fresh.

Bears and Drugs

The use of anabolic steroids by bears is less noticeable and less talked about than in other gay groups, because of the fact that many bears are naturally built big, and because people in general assume that bears are not concerned with body image. This, as Jay's story proves, is not always true. In some cases, aspiring muscle bears will use anabolic steroids to build their otherwise naturally lean or high-fat physiques. Anabolic steroid use is one of the less known little secrets of bear culture. In bear culture, just like with other subcultures, anabolic steroids have gained popularity out of a concern for body image.

Steroid use in bear culture is less shocking than it really seems. A fallacy is that bears are really unaffected by body image.

If bear culture was not susceptible to body image, the muscle bear would not have the superstar status among bears that it enjoys today. There are now many competitions around the world for Mr. Bear titles. One has to question just how this is different from the objectification of men that bears criticize. The rise of the muscle bear in bear culture is a loud statement that the jolly old bear on which the culture was based could be improved, that he can become more masculine, more muscled, a sexier and more desirable bear.

It is understandable why some older bears feel uncomfortable about the rise of the muscled bear. For many of them, muscle bears are the anomaly of bear culture. But that is exactly what makes it interesting, that the muscle bear is both the end product of bear culture and at the same a threat to it. He represents the future of bear culture as much as he represents a threat to its founding values.

> Boy, it's [muscle bear phenomenon] booming! But I just see it and I don't relate to it, I think it sets up a hierarchy, a super bear. . . . My partner and I were in Florida, and we went to something called the Wolf Fest, and it was like this bear beauty contest and I don't understand it. That is not where the roots were—the roots were against that.[15]

This situation opens up the door for one to play devil's advocate and pose some questions: What happens to bear culture if the gym becomes a focal point or pastime for bears? If bears get very muscular and/or lean and they no longer look like bears, what happens then? Can you still be a bear if you no longer look like one?

To be a muscle bear built by free weights is, after all, more time consuming and complicated than just being a bear. If we ask what it takes to be a muscle bear, the list includes serious and sometimes daily workouts, high-calorie and protein diets, and in many cases, even the bear unthinkable: trimming of body hair. Interestingly enough, because muscle bears are more aesthetically influenced, body and facial hair are often neatly trimmed. In a nutshell, being a muscle bear takes time, money, and dedication—like being a circuit boy or an athlete or a fashionista. More important, it takes an emotional and social connection to the group around which the subculture revolves, its unspecified dynamics, and adherence to its implicit rules and regulations.

All bears are not created equal, and neither are their points of view. Although Luke enjoys being a muscle bear because of the attention he receives, he feels that in some ways the muscle bear ideal "does a disservice" to bears, that "it's another way of separating people. I don't think it's healthy for the guys who may never be able to look like that."[16] A newbie to bearness, Jay had a rude awakening to Luke's concerns just last year:

> We found ourselves in conflict last year at Lazy Bear up at the river. We wound up camping at the Willows for the weekend, my boyfriend Mark and myself and another friend. And apparently most of the guys that were staying at the Willows were not part of the party scene, or of the muscle bears. They were just, you know, big, fat bears. Some of them didn't get out of their lawn chairs all day, they never left the Willows. It's this group that goes back every year, and they all knew each other, and we were the outsiders. We had no idea this was like that. They didn't like us.[17]
>
> We went out and partied—no one else there went out or partied—they all visited and did the whole camping thing like you'd expect straight people camping, just socializing. I mean nothing is wrong with that, but we didn't fit in. We were like outcasts—when we came back from FAB [a Russian River nightclub], Mark and I had sex in our tent at night, and everyone is clearing their throats all night and telling us to be quiet, which is hard when you're camping next to each other. If we had been with muscle bears or people who partied a little more, it wouldn't have been like that. They would have probably tried to come in instead (laughs). So that was interesting, and I became aware of some of the differences.

When I ask Jay if he thinks that partying by muscle bears is splitting bear culture between the bears who party and those who do not, he thinks that it does, and agrees that its more likely for a muscle bear to party than for a regular bear:

> The bears who party are in better shape, it's just like the rest of gay culture: the guys who go out and party and go to circuit events, they are in better shape. I think it's a trickle-down effect into this bear culture.

Jay makes an interesting point about the trickle-down effect from mainstream gay culture's concern with body image and aesthetics.

While it is too soon to predict that another subculture will emerge based on the concept of the "circuit bear," the suggestion is not too far-fetched. Today, in San Francisco, one of the most visible assemblies of bears is a group of about fifty (and growing) muscle bears who like to meet up and go out clubbing, and have formed a group appropriately titled The Dancing Bears.

Bears are at the gym mainly out of an influential concern for body image. In my survey there was a direct correlation between those who were satisfied with their body and those who were the most muscle bound. Bears often indicated dissatisfaction with their bodies, but muscle bears as a group were much more satisfied than those who identified only as bears, though not as satisfied as bodybuilders or athletes. Given the powerful influence that the muscle bear and its ideal image has achieved in such a short time, it gives us a glance into the future of what is now a muscle-bound bear culture.

THE MUSCLE BEAR PARADOX

Bear culture as a social group is so new that it is difficult to write about it with great conviction—the group as a whole keeps undergoing changes. In spite of this, the popularity of beardom as a social trend indicates that bear culture is not just here to stay, but that it will continue to grow into an enduring and powerful cultural subgroup.

Bears and muscle bears continue teaching us about bear culture. But in the two decades that bear culture has been around it has vacillated between the renunciation of one standard body image to the idealization of another. It has gone from condemning underwear models to worshiping its own version of the male supermodel, from avoiding the extremes of being body conscious to the inclusion of steroids into the equation, and last (and most entertaining perhaps), from organizing dinner parties and picnics to adopting the modus operandi of the circuit to produce social events.

The muscle bear is somewhat of an anomaly. The previously mentioned inconsistencies might be interesting and entertaining at best, and for the most part, verge on the trivial. Bear culture cannot be best described in black and white terms. Subcultures in general are socially complex and multidimensional; with this in mind, let's take a closer look at a very important and less trivial matter that the muscle bear has brought to the surface of gay culture: the fitness and health of bears.

BEAR FITNESS AND HEALTH

To fitness, health, and mental professionals, bear culture represents an interesting dilemma. From a health perspective, bear culture has both desirable and undesirable traits.

On the one hand, here is an entire subculture built around men whose acceptance of their bodies is commendable. This is, for the average American, a very difficult thing to do, and it is something that fitness professionals and psychologists spend much of their careers on: teaching clients and patients to love and accept their bodies.

On the other hand, in light of the serious health implications of being overweight and/or obese, there is a problem with an entire subculture that goes beyond accepting obesity: they idealize it. Although illicit drug abuse is not rampant in bear culture, alcoholism is, and so is heart disease, diabetes, high blood pressure, and all of the other ailments that are associated with obesity. From a medical perspective, like a circuit boy abusing drugs, an obese bear overindulging in food and alcohol is a heart-attack-waiting-to-happen. The only difference is in the substances.

In bear culture there is a small group of men who call themselves "growers," people who aspire to get as fat and as big as they can, sometimes to the extent of immobility. This is the other side of eating disorders and negative body image that does not get talked about much, and one which I will not discuss at length because, as with other eating and body image disorders, it makes up only a tiny segment of the population.

From a health perspective, the implications of ignoring the body altogether pose a lethal threat to bears and to bear culture. What bear culture needs is a healthy medium in which large but healthy are interchangeable. Simply put, if bears do not take care of their bodies, our furry friends will become an endangered species. I am happy to report that in today's gay gym culture, a growing number of bears and muscle bears, including Jay and Luke, are striving for this concept. Muscle bears often represent a younger generation of bears who are trying to find a happy medium in gay culture, and we can learn a lot from them. They are teaching us that there can be a balance between bear and gay cultures, between inactivity and fitness, and between standard beauty ideals that don't include them and those created by them.

In discussing the role of health and aesthetics in modern gay culture, our strongman, Luke, tells us what motivates him and his relationship with body image and the misconception that to be healthy one needs to be thin:

> I think it's really important to be healthy. Would I like to be thin and muscular like you? I would, but to do that I'd have to have surgery. . . . So, am I healthy? Yes, I am healthy. I'm forty-seven years old; my blood pressure is 120 over 70 most of the time, I've had HIV for nineteen years, I should be dead, and I am not. I'm a world champion athlete. Am I thin? No.[18]

I predict that the influx of bear culture into the gym will, over time, have a balancing effect on gay body culture in general. By the same token, the injecting of a healthy dose of gym culture into bear culture is sure to reshape and somewhat restructure the subgroup. The growing presence of muscle bears at the gym and in different forms of media sends a strong message to other gay men: you can be healthy and sexy without six-pack abs. For those for whom a six-pack is next to impossible or not that important, that message is a big relief. In essence, these groups can learn from each other: while bears can learn to shape and build their bodies from muscle boys, muscle boys can learn from bears to love and accept their bodies.

Ideals of beauty and reality are often two very different things. Bear culture, for all its complexities and contradictions, might hold the solution we all need to arrive at a healthy balance between aesthetics and health and between ideals and reality. Now, that's a concept worthy of a big-bear-hug.

Chapter 11

The Older Male

Lenny Simpson

Leonard (Lenny) A. Simpson (a pseudonym) is a fifty-eight-year-old orthopedic surgeon who lives in San Francisco. An active member in the gay community, Lenny can be found at charity events, athletic events, parties, and occasionally at one of the local dance clubs or circuit parties. But one place Lenny visits every day is the gym. He has been working out for about thirty years. "Working out is a primary concern," he says. "It is one of my highest priorities."

> [working out] made me feel better about myself and increased my self-esteem. It made me feel better about my appearance. It made me, I think, more alert. It helped with insomnia. It gave me a social outlet to relate to people on a good level.[1]

Lenny's dedication to fitness has paid off: his body looks lean and hard, and he is without doubt in better physical shape than many of the twenty-five-year-olds at the gym. Lenny's body doesn't just look good: he can more than carry his own weight, literally and figuratively. I first met Lenny while we were both on the California AIDS Ride. In the years since, I've watched Lenny train for several swimming competitions and triathlons.

The "older male," which in the medical community is typically defined as those above age forty, makes up one of the largest and fastest-growing segments of gay gym culture. This group is primarily made up of the Baby Boomer generation, as the youngest boomers are now in their mid- to late forties, (a smaller portion are in their golden years). When gay men reach the forty-year milestone, the reasons they go to the gym start to multiply. Looking good is still important,

Muscle Boys: Gay Gym Culture
Published by The Haworth Press, Taylor & Francis Group, 2008.
doi:10.1300/6034_11

and so is the socialization that gay men enjoy at the gym, but health management and disease prevention become more significant. For older gay men, staying healthy is more important than aesthetics and can mean the difference between health and disease, independent living and assisted living, and ultimately life and death.

HEALTH

Although most Baby Boomers have enjoyed their status as members of the largest-ever U.S. generation, gay Baby Boomers were shaken by the worst plague of modern history. From the early 1980s to the early 1990s, during the peak of the AIDS epidemic in the United States, a huge number of gay boomers died of AIDS, and those who survived often watched their friends and lovers die more frequently and painfully than seemed possible. In gay America, the number of men lost to the epidemic vastly diminished the size of the group.

Michael Meehan (Chapter 5) discussed what it was like to work out at gay gyms back in 1978. However, when I interviewed him, his first sentence was not about the gyms, but about his lost peers:

> The worst part is that I don't see the guys around anymore. The ones who were big and buff, the most attractive, are the ones who went the fastest. It was this terrible irony of seeing guys who had achieved perfection, and then you see them in the street a few weeks later, rapidly gone. They would go in six months. I feel like I lost a frame of reference, when I look around for other men my age who are working out just to know where do I go from here. Where's my role model? Who do I look for at this age, to know what I'm going to look like in five years or what I'm capable of in five years? There's no one there, I mean there is just no one. They all died.[2]

A fifty-year-old HIV-positive man in New York City who took my survey and who identifies as a bodybuilder wrote:

> One thing important is to understand how seeing all of your lovers die over a couple of decades has made a lot of us very self-reliant and into serious bodybuilding as a means for trying to deal with the hideous side effects of HIV drugs . . .

Those who survived the worst of the epidemic, like Michael, and those who are personally fighting it, like the fifty-year-old New Yorker, are not ignorant of the importance of health. Because of this, as well as the wisdom gained with age, gay Baby Boomers and seniors have become one of the principal segments of gay gym culture. When it comes to the gym, one of the main differences between older gay men and their younger counterparts is that the older ones are understandably much more concerned with their health.

Thirty-three percent (1,838) of the men who took my survey make up the over-forty/older male group, (second in size only to the muscle boy category), and the majority of these older men, 27 percent (1,517) of total survey respondents, range in age between forty and fifty years old. When I asked the question: "What are your reasons for working out and your involvement with the gym?" the older male survey respondents provided me the majority of answers correlating health to involvement with the gym. Over 1,000 responses in my survey from older gay men were similar to these:

> Diabetes and heart condition.
> (Sixty-one-year-old from Massachusetts)
>
> Therapy for back and spine.
> (A forty-seven-year-old, Canada)
>
> Keeping a healthy heart.
> (A retired sixty-four-year-old from Arizona)
>
> Had sleep apnea and needed to lose weight.
> (Forty-five-year-old from New York City)
>
> Diet and exercise reduced my cholesterol from 300 to 174. My overall health has dramatically improved.
> (Fifty-two-year-old from California)
>
> I have had heart disease for eight years now and it has helped me to keep healthy. Basically it was: work out or drop dead.
> (A forty-eight-year-old in Wisconsin)

As men approach middle age, the difference in how we look and how we feel differs dramatically compared with our younger years.

Many older men become concerned that their bodies have already weakened and aged. Many start losing their hair, others simply cannot fit into those favorite jeans anymore, yet others notice that the grocery bags they used to carry with ease start feeling much heavier. The value of being fit becomes ever more apparent.

John Amodio is a sixty-three-year-old in San Francisco. He has been working out since 1997:

> I think back in 1997 it was for other reasons, I think I got caught up in the culture of wanting to have a fine looking body, to be more appealing, to attract men, etc. And then that has evolved over the years for other priorities, and it's now health reasons . . . I am a diabetic, I have had open heart surgery, I have just recently been diagnosed with high blood pressure, and working out was not always been easy, I kind of got into a rut . . . but since I started working out with a personal trainer for the first time I've seen results in my physique, in how I feel, and more importantly the medical numbers, the hemoglobin AC1 test is a better number, the cholesterol is a better number, and we are working on the high blood pressure. The results I've seen are the biggest motivator, and I want to go further, I want to see more results physically and medically.[3]

A common concern shared by younger and older gay men alike when it comes to the gym is aesthetics. But as the body ages, health enters the equation.

> Just the process of getting older and living with a body that's fighting gravity and age, knowing that there is lower back stiffness, and shoulder stiffness, and hip stiffness, and risk of osteoporosis make me aware of the health benefits of working out as well as the aesthetics of it.
>
> So, if there is a day that I don't feel motivated to go to the gym it may be the health benefits that motivate me more than the aesthetics. I can very well see that for a younger person it may be only the aesthetics, because they have not confronted the issues of aging.[4]

Muscle Loss with Aging

After about age thirty, it's estimated that the average man loses up to seven pounds of muscle every ten years. When we're young, our muscles possess enough strength to make effortless what the medical field has termed activities of daily living (ADL): walking across a room, typing at a keyboard, bringing a coffee cup to our lips. During adolescence, muscles and other tissue (bones and joints) as well as the organs mature whether you're working out or not (although muscles in particular tend to become more developed when physical activity is added). As it ages, the body slowly loses its ability to synthesize and maintain lean mass on its own. If we lose enough muscle mass—and the majority of older men who do not exercise do—we lose the firmness and shape the muscles provide for the body, and along with that goes the stability, structural support, and command in executing ADL. At this point, simple things such as walking upstairs, getting up from the toilet, and carrying a grocery bag will start to become difficult—and in some cases, eventually impossible.

The myth that muscle can turn into fat may have evolved from the fact that as people get older they grow fatter and lose their muscle tone, giving the illusion that the muscle has turned into fat. This is impossible: muscle and fat are two completely different types of tissue. What has occurred is that the muscles have shrunk and the amount of fat has increased.

The two most efficient and natural methods for managing body fat are nutrition and exercise. Healthy individuals can control how much weight they gain or lose and how much fat is stored in their bodies by exercising and eating sensibly. As far as nutrition goes, the types, and more importantly, the amounts of food we eat determine just how much fat gets stored and how much gets used. This is the role of healthy and balanced eating. Through exercise we can control fat in two ways: (1) by burning calories through exercise activity, and (2) by maintaining lean muscle which, because of its energy demands, consumes more calories than fat does.

The muscle-fat relationship works like this: The body's survival mechanisms (homeostasis), which are controlled by the brain, effectively maintain the body's total weight. So, what occurs on a metabolic level is that as the body loses muscle weight, the brain's red light mechanism goes off, and in an effort to ensure the body's survival (by maintaining body weight), the brain signals the body to store extra calories, regardless of where these calories come from. The body's metabolic system then stores extra calories in the form of—you guessed it—fat.

The Skinny on Fat

It has been said that men work out to build muscle because you cannot flex fat, and like other overused clichés, there is a lot of truth to this one. Structurally speaking, fat is flaccid tissue, which explains why it has earned the names "blubber" and "flab." Despite its bad reputation, fat is necessary: it provides the body with insulation because the body stores fat under the skin (subcutaneous adipose tissue) in addition to the physiologically *essential fat,*[5] which is stored in bone marrow, brain, spinal cord, and other internal organs. Fat also assists with metabolism and provides another extremely important resource: energy. Energy comes from the foods we eat (carbohydrates, fat, protein), and fat provides about half of the calories for daily living.

Fat is measured on the body as a percentage of body weight. Desired body fat for optimum health in males is around 15 to 18 percent depending on age and other factors. Of this number, only 3 to 4 percent make up essential fat, the rest pads the body mostly in the form of subcutaneous fat, and in the case of very overweight and obese individuals, intramuscular (within the muscle) fat as well. Although fat is important in the human body, in males, 15 percent is more than plenty for all of the body's needs, plus enough to run a marathon or two. Athletes and bodybuilders have lower percentages of body fat.

Because fat is so necessary, the body stores it for future use. Regardless of where calories came from (carbohydrates, fat, or protein), excess calories are stored in the form of body fat. This storage process is very important in humans because the stored fat will later provide energy for everything we do (working, walking, moving, etc.), and even the energy to sustain the body when we are not doing anything (such as sitting on the sofa or sleeping). At rest, about 50 percent of the calories that the human body uses come from stored fat. This fat-storage mechanism is vital to sustaining life—but, as we all know, too much of a good thing is, well, not a good thing.

The difference should be made between having a few pounds of body fat here and there and having an excess amount. Men who have more than 20 percent of their body weight in fat are categorized as overweight, and when the reading is 30 percent or higher they are considered obese. Excess fat creates more work for the body, not just by slowing it down as it is more work to carry around extra weight, but also because metabolizing fat takes much more energy (about twice as much) as metabolizing other fuels (like carbohydrates and protein), which, in the long run, forces the heart and other organs to work overtime. Being overfat taxes our bodies into disease.

It is now estimated (by numerous sources) that about 30 percent of Americans are obese, a figure that amounts to roughly 75 million people. This is concerning because the diseases associated with being overly fat largely make up the roster of major killers in the United States: heart disease, high blood pressure, diabetes, etc. In addition, obesity correlates with other less threatening yet serious conditions such as osteoporosis, decreased energy, stress, depression, sexual dysfunction, and isolation to name a few.

Other Health Issues

When it comes to exercise, in terms of body aesthetics, preserving youth really translates into maintaining the firmness of our bodies—preserving our muscles. In doing this, we also maintain other aspects of health that correlate with being young: leanness, more energy, less taxed organs and biological systems (cardiovascular, digestive, etc.). In addition, in men, exercising on a regular basis will promote the body's synthesis of testosterone, thereby stimulating the male sexual drive.

As an older male and a physician, Lenny Simpson does not have to be sold on the idea of working out. He understands well that exercise has plenty of benefits besides staving off weight gain:

> Oh, there is no doubt . . . of the strong medical aspects of it. There is no doubt that osteoporosis increases with aging and inactivity, and one of the things that can really combat osteoporosis is weight-bearing exercise, weight lifting. There is also a tendency for major joints to become more immobile as you age, resulting in a decreased range of motion, and working out and stretching can combat that as well. Also, working out helps to produce a mental alertness that people who don't exercise may not have.[6]

Another debilitating weakness that comes with the onset of older age is the loss of bone density that can result in osteoporosis. The weakened structural system resulting from osteoporosis makes it more difficult for older adults to have commanding stability; it also makes it very easy for the bones to break with a fall on the sidewalk that would not seriously hurt a younger and stronger healthy person. Because the bones are weak, the recovery process can be long, difficult, and painful. Many older adults never truly recover from a fall. The immobility adds to the complications of old age coupled with disease. Though osteoporosis is a more common ailment among older females, the disease nonetheless affects many men as well. Besides medication, weight training is one of the best antidotes to osteoporosis, as weight-bearing exercise will increase bone density and strengthen the bones.

Managing body weight via exercise and nutrition can greatly affect how we manage other aging issues such as decreased mobility, diabetes, and high blood pressure. I've had clients who were able to go off of blood pressure medication completely once they lost twenty pounds of excess fat and got in better shape. Likewise, a more effective metabolism aids diabetes patients in blood glucose management, as well as better digestion and more efficient absorption of medications to manage not just diabetes but many other medical conditions. Exercise and sound nutrition, for the older adult, are nothing short of a win-win situation.

Exercise has become such an important ingredient in the management of aging that recently, in medical and academic circles, the term Sedentary Death Syndrome (SeDS) has been coined and increasingly used to describe the results in disease as a byproduct of inactivity by older adults.[7]

INDEPENDENT LIVING

Cecil Franco (a pseudonym), seventy-nine, is a retired professor who was born in the Midwest and has spent most of his adult life living in San Francisco. He didn't start going to the gym until his late sixties when, at the advice of his doctor, he made a trip to the local health club and signed up. "I clearly went for health reasons; I didn't have a chronic illness, but I was overweight."[8]

Cecil has been a regular at the gym ever since, and a couple of years ago he became one of my clients. In the time we have been training together, he has become stronger, and his balance and mobility have improved.

Not only is Cecil in great shape for someone his age, he is often in better shape than people young enough to be his grandchildren. Not too long ago, he had to slow down to wait for an out-of-shape colleague in her thirties who was having a much harder time going up the stairs. Though he was still teaching (he retired at seventy-eight), he often had to slow down and wait for the students to catch up to him on the stairs. "They were just out shape . . . a lot of them would rather take the elevator because the stairs were quite difficult for them."

Cecil's involvement with the gym and the level of fitness he has acquired have given him a certain level of confidence not always typical of seventy-nine-year-olds:

> I've realized that age doesn't have to become an absolute barrier. Even though I'm older there are many physical things I can do and in some way even do better than some younger people.[9]

When asked about his fitness goals, Cecil is very clear: "Independent living: that's one of my goals."

> I like to be able to decide what I want to do and when I want to do it. Privacy has always been an important element in my life. But as you grow older you realize that you may not be able to exercise your independence. Now that I'm retired, I realize that I can have a lot of independence. I want to be strong enough to be able to carry the groceries up the stairs and all the other things. And to be sexually active—I want to be in good enough physical condition so I can keep having the sex. Indeed, the sex is very enjoyable to me . . .

Like Cecil, more older gay men are joining their local gyms to be involved in their health management, and their results are astonishing:

> I used to think of my body as evil and unhealthy. I didn't feel I belonged in the gym. I don't have that feeling now; I think of myself of being reasonably healthy for my age. I never thought of myself as physically skilled in any way whatsoever, and go-

> ing to the gym has changed that. I can actually lift the weights! I can actually bend parts of my body that I thought were fixed for life. So the body has become more manageable; more useful; something not to fear but to use and to value.[10]

Scientific research on strength training in eighty-year-olds has shown up to 200 percent increases in strength. What does this mean? Well, for a reasonably healthy thirty-year-old a 200 percent increase in strength is usually only noticeable at the gym and in the size of his pecs. For an eighty-year-old it can mean that he can walk again, get out of a chair without help, and use the toilet unassisted. It means that he can walk to the store, carry his grocery bag home, and cook himself a meal. Simply put, it can mean the difference between feeling content and productive or feeling helpless and dependent. Needless to say, fitness can have a profound effect on an older person's quality of life.

STEROIDS AND THE OLDER MALE

More often than not, older men who use anabolic steroids have a prescription and their physicians closely monitor their health. As I have discussed earlier in this book, the most common reason for taking the prescribed drugs is hypogonadism or low levels of testosterone—a condition that becomes more and more common as men get older. What is new to the medical territory is the added concern in regard to body image by older men—especially gay men.

I have a friend in his early seventies who works out three or four times a week. At his request, his doctor has, over the past few years, prescribed him several anabolic steroids, including testosterone, Deca Durabolin, and human growth hormone—requests the doctor did not question given his low testosterone levels as revealed by blood tests. As a result of the training and the drugs, his body looks more like that of a fit thirty-five-year-old, and his energy and sex drive rival that of a vivacious twenty-something.

Like my friend in his seventies, a lot of men are finding out that anabolic steroids can have a huge effect not just on body composition, but on sex drive, energy, and other quality-of-life issues. The issue is one that physicians are meeting head on. As Dr. Moller told me:

> Doctors do similar things for women who are undergoing the natural process of menopause, with estrogen supplementation. Part of the reason it has been justified is to prevent bone loss, but part of it also is that some women really have severe mental changes as the hormonal levels are changing. So, analogous to that it is the thought that, well, men have some of those changes, not as quickly but more chronically, so maybe we should be supplementing men who are in their sixties and seventies with [anabolic steroids, especially testosterone] and getting them feeling better. [11]

Hormone replacement therapy (HRT) for men is becoming a more common practice, especially in dense and sophisticated urban centers. As a forty-nine-year-old from Los Angeles who took my survey wrote:

> Two years ago, my doctor put me on hormone replacement therapy, which involves the use of the anabolic steroid Depo-Testosterone. The prescription is for a very small amount and is nowhere near the quantity that professional bodybuilders use. The primary effects are improved self-confidence, increased body hair (had none before I started, now have a hairy chest and stomach), and a major increase in sex drive. The idea is that your testosterone level should be restored to the level it was when you were twenty-five years old. The HRT does not involve any other anabolic steroids or growth hormone. However, I now know that if I did use those other drugs, I would be much bigger than I am today, and the whole campaign about "steroids are BAD for you" is a complete lie and a failure. The HRT program is proof that when these drugs are used properly, there are tremendous benefits.

Given the complex implications of steroid use, even by older men who clearly benefit from them medically, the situation creates not just a medical dilemma, but also a moral one. For one, the drugs pose potential health risks; also, since they are a controlled substance, there is a moral implication against their use. Whether an older man is prescribed steroids is unfortunately a decision influenced not by medical protocol but more often than not by a collective "moral modus operandi" that looks down on the drugs.

In a candid discussion, I brought up the fact that when the patient is a healthy seventy-year-old whose life expectancy is seventy-five, the dialogue ought to change. At that point in his life, the patient will most likely not live long enough to be negatively affected by the potential risks involved in anabolic therapy. Does it not make sense then to weigh risks against benefits? Medically speaking, are these not the symptoms the drugs were designed to alleviate in the first place? Should we gamble on quality of life during those last few years at the cost of trivial moral values and medical ignorance?

Of course, these questions are easier for me to ask than for a practicing physician to decide on:

> It's a process of weighing the situation. If they are seventy and they have a lot of fatigue and not much sex drive at all, and maybe they're having trouble maintaining erections and maybe they're feeling bad about themselves. It's kind of like, well, so you might increase their risk a little bit of cardiac complications . . . is it worth it to prescribe it? And I'm sure there are some physicians now who are weighing that balance. I don't necessarily think it's a bad thing to be doing for older men, although the medical establishment still strongly does view it as something that shouldn't be done, and I think some of course put themselves out there at risk of being reprimanded by the medical community if they do something too far outside the realms of normal medical practice. . . .[12]

Never mind that "normal medical practice" is in this case far from scientifically sound and instead often dictated by uninformed moral decorum. However, even with the odds against the practice, steroid use by older men is a growing trend, one that I predict will only gain momentum. At that point, I hope, there will be some sound research and better-informed medical decisions.

AESTHETICS, DATING, AND THE ATTRACTIVE OLDER MALE

Because men are much more muscular than women, muscle is associated with maleness. To a great extent the male musculature is part of the social mask that illustrates our manhood. The amount of muscle on men is directly proportional to brute male power, force, strength, and vigor. Because throughout millennia man has had to depend on sway and might to survive, the importance attached to musculature is understandable. This further explains our romantic and sexual attachment to the sturdy, well-developed male.

The association has entertained the minds of men from the times of Plato to Darwin. Darwin, of course, refined and popularized the theory, and now modern scientists and more specifically genetic research has concluded that the desire for men to be muscular and the physical attraction of potential mates (both gay men and straight women) toward muscular men is simply hardwired into us.[13]

When a man is very muscular, he is described as brawny, studly, strong, and virile to name a few; when he is not, he is often referred to as scrawny, weak, and by association feminine. In direct contrast, what defines traditional beautiful bodies in females is the curvaceous hourglass figure, shaped by the heavy concentration of fatty tissue that makes up much of the breasts and hips. On the other hand, when a woman is very muscular she is said to appear manly, and many find her unattractive. Although these definitions and their associations are slowly changing, and we are seeing more positive associations to a leaner and more muscular female body, we must remember that this is a twenty-first-century phenomenon that is only in its beginning stages.

Besides feeling better, John Amodio tells me that he is also looking better:

> I'm a little more defined. I've noticed an increased availability of men more frequently that I had in the past. I'm going to the same places that I used to, but since I've taken on the training and have more definition on my body and less weight, people seek me out, which is a nice thing. I've found that to be a positive side effect of the effort that I've put into exercise.
>
> Every morning, when I finish a shower, I have this routine, the way my house is set up, I go into a small bedroom right off the bathroom and I usually dry off there and I have these double mirrors and I just take a moment and look. And now, when I do, I can see the difference, I can see shape, I can see definition, I can see lean, the waistline has been reduced, and I can also see

> that in the clothes, that makes me feel good. And that in the morning, getting up and having that reaction to yourself, to look at yourself that way inward, it makes me feel good. And that positive self-image does wonders in other aspects of your life . . . just going out to work and going out the door, you feel good, you have a skip to your walk.[14]

The aesthetic concerns of older gay men are very much like those of younger ones: looking leaner and more muscular, attracting mates, looking good. But working out can have a more dramatic aesthetic effect on an aging body than on a younger one. This is because very often, younger people are in shape just because they are young, not because they work out. But by weight training and eating sensibly, men cannot only reverse the muscle loss and fat gain that occurs with aging, they can often become more muscular and leaner than they were when they were younger. I have over and over again heard older men say "I'm in better shape now at forty (or fifty) than I was at twenty (or thirty)."

I've shared a locker room with Rick Dinihanian for years, and we eventually became friends, but even before I knew him it was hard not to notice his body. His bulging pecs, ripped six-pack, rounded biceps, and bubble butt suggest all the classic features of a *Playgirl* model—with one exception: the silver hair, courtesy of his fifty-seven years. In June of 2004, Rick made waves in the media by becoming, at fifty-five, the oldest ever centerfold and cover model to grace the pages of *Playgirl,* and since then he's become not just a spokesmodel for men his age, but solid proof that older and hot are not mutually exclusive. Rick's *Playgirl* experience, including his subsequent magazine and television interviews, was so life altering that he made a midlife career switch. After moving from San Francisco to New York City he continued to model. In addition, as a response to hundreds of letters and e-mails requesting his secret to staying fit, Rick opened a private core strength and fitness studio in Manhattan where he has trained such celebrities as Jessica Lange, Rosanne Cash, and Harry Hamlin.

Older gay men, like Rick Dinihanian, in impressive numbers, are proving wrong the misconception that as we age, our bodies just go to hell. As I have discussed widely in other chapters, most guys half his age go to the gym because they want a body that looks like Rick's.

As Lenny told me:

> The myth that's been changing in the gay community is that there is no place socially or culturally for the older gay male, that the older gay male is not a vibrant, healthy, sexual being. I think that well-toned older gay men are now seen visually as vibrant sexual beings, and this is destroying some of the myths that tend to discard the older person.[15]

Younger people tend to disregard the older male as nonsexual. But Lenny Simpson, John Amodio, and Rick Dinihanian have proved them wrong. In response to my survey, a forty-eight-year-old from Washington, DC, wrote that when it comes to working out and staying physically fit, "As a post-40s GWM, it curbs a bit of the feeling of diminishing return of attractiveness and attentiveness." A forty-one-year-old from San Diego wrote that exercise has "Kept me healthy, boosted my self-esteem, and reduced stress levels. And it clearly has both raised and prolonged my sexual marketability."

Very much like their younger counterparts, the older gay male is largely motivated to work out to be more attractive to potential mates. Many are single and on the dating/sex market well into their fifties, sixties, and seventies. Many are not single, but in open relationships, so technically speaking still "on the sex market." Invariably, the shape and firmness of the body is still a significant factor in the mating process of older males.

A forty-one-year-old from New Jersey wrote:

> Up until age thirty-three I was always skinny and very average. I'm in much better shape at forty-one than I was at eighteen or twenty-five and it feels great. I'm pretty shy, so being in shape tends to make people more receptive to me, both in business and in a social scene. Getting compliments feels good, too, and makes working out even more rewarding. It also encourages an all-around healthy lifestyle for me. I rarely drink, never do drugs, eat reasonably well (though there's plenty of room for improvement) and basically wake up every morning excited to start the day.

A forty-four-year-old bisexual man in California wrote that working out replaced his "low self-esteem" and that it has influenced his body image:

> I love how I look, I get tons of compliments and it motivates me. Working out has given me the confidence to go out in the world and get anything I want. It has totally changed my life and who I am. Men and woman are always chasing me around—it's hot!

Sexuality is an important factor for why older gay men desire to stay in shape. When asked about peer pressure, Lenny tells us that "I personally have a lover who's twenty-five years my junior; I feel some pressure to keep my looks and my tone up to be attractive for him."

A lot of men, unfortunately, give up on the presumed (and faulty) assumption that they are too old to be attractive—or sexual for that matter. In men, biology dictates that men can be sexual and even father children well into their seventies and even eighties. The notion that older men are not sexual is more an ageism-based social construction than a biologically determined consequence. It is a distressing reality, but many older men stop having sex because they give up, not because they are older. It is often these same men who will typically use the same "I'm too old" excuse for everything else. As Cecil tells us: "It's part of this stereotype that as you get older you have to grow more and more disabled. There is some reality to that, but people use it as an excuse for not exercising."

Self-Confidence

In his book *Life Outside,* Michelangelo Signorile's portrayal of the "lonely old queen" would have us believe that all gay men past forty who go to the gym are not just desperate but delusional.[16] This is simply not true. The majority of older gay men who are involved in the gym are quite comfortable with who they are and what they look like. These men clearly make an effort to look good at their age, but with a few exceptions they are not spending ten hours a week at the gym to train for the next circuit party. In both surveys I conducted (the one in San Francisco gyms and the one online) and in just about every interview that I did, those older men who exercise on a regular basis will report more confidence and better self-image than those who do not.

In many cases, the older we get, the more our relationship to our own aesthetics and how we define aesthetics changes. As Cecil points out:

> I've always had a peculiar relationship to my body. I've never thought of myself as being . . . physically present. When I started working out, I was already an older male. I wanted to get rid of the fat, and wanted to be thin. And yes, I guess I wanted to be more attractive within the limitations I have to work with, but never went very far in that direction. You know, you have to be realistic about these things . . .[17]

Culturally speaking, the "muscle daddy" has become as much an object of desire as his younger counterparts. For one, often the maturity that also sets in with aging results in the development of a better self-image, an attractive attribute on its own. Furthermore, as Rick Dinihanian told me, he doesn't just get second glances on the street or in the locker room—he gets fan mail. And the mail comes both from men his age, and men young enough to be his grandchildren. Technically, these hot older guys have no reason to envy the younger jocks. In fact, sometimes it is the younger jocks who cannot compete with the older ones! As a fifty-six-year-old from West Virginia who identifies as a "Muscle Bear," and a "Daddy," wrote that he is "Fascinated by the expanding interest of young men in men my age."

Social critics tend to diminish the importance of exercise in the health management of an aging population. This is not only socially irresponsible—it is unacceptable. The difficulties associated with an aging body are no laughing matter. Aging men need encouragement, not criticism or critics making fun of their efforts. A regular exercise program provides much leverage toward independent and happy lifestyles and nothing short of such should be encouraged.

SOCIAL OUTLET

One of the most remarkable differences between gay men and straight men is easily observed in the lifestyles they lead. The near nonexistence of traditional marriages and children bestow gay men as a group with higher disposable incomes and more free time than their straight male counterparts. To a great extent, the prevalence of gay gym culture, as well as other time-demanding organizations popular in the gay world, are largely the result of this cultural phenomenon.

Social venues and opportunities often, however, diminish as gay men get older, and this lack of social outlets has become a problem.

As members of our community start approaching their sixties, seventies, and eighties, they retire from their jobs, and their partners, relatives, and friends start to die, often leaving the older person in social isolation. The isolation problem is further fueled by health ailments that often limit the older person's mobility. The disconnection from the rest of the world can then lead to a lack of proper health care and often, psychological (depression, anxiety, etc.) as well physical health problems. A recent study by Brian Heaphy at Nottingham Trent University determined that among other complexities of aging, older gay men often feel isolated and excluded.[18]

When I asked John Amodio if the gym replaced anything in his life he is quick to answer: "Boredom. There was a period prior to when I didn't go to the gym when there was nothing. I didn't have any other activities."[19]

Even for gay men in their thirties and forties, who are not near retirement, the social scene starts to contract. As Lenny points out:

> I'm a person who does not do well in a bar scene, I don't like the effects of alcohol. The gym allows me to pursue an activity and perhaps make social contact with a hello or a conversation in a non-threatening, safe environment. In today's day and age with the Internet it can be very difficult to have human contact, and the gym allows that in a balanced way. For me it's an excellent social outlet.[20]

In American urban areas there are limited social outlets for older gay men such as gay and lesbian community centers. Places and organizations such as these occasionally offer older gay men seminars, workshops, and other social programs. These programs are often quite successful, showing the demand for social outlets for older gay men in dense urban areas. However, the majority of these events, even in places like San Francisco and New York City, are often too far apart and too random to truly be an ongoing support system, and this is a problem. Even worse, when we get outside of the urban gay ghetto environment, social outlets for older gay men decrease dramatically (to nonexistence sometimes) and are more often than not reduced to the local gay bar, if there is one.

Facing our own mortality is a difficult thing to do at any age, but those of us who are still young do the task quite poorly. Most of us are the result of an American culture that is very youth-oriented, and the subject of aging, like that of death, is not only unbecoming but is held in reserve for the old, not for the young. In America, aging is a taboo subject, an undefined anti-American ideal. And in the gay world, ageism seems to multiply. Gay media and a good majority of social events, like circuit parties, are youth oriented. Ageism in gay America is one of the biggest and most largely unnoticed yet destructive problems of our time.

The effects of ageism on gay men result in isolation from the rest of the community. The isolation then results in a series of social, mental, and health-related problems. There is very little, if any, interaction between groups of younger and older gay men. Unlike the traditional nuclear heterosexual family in which young and old make up daily life as well as holidays, modern gay lifestyles in middle age revolve much more around friends, co-workers, and lovers of a similar age group. Furthermore, as it is in straight society, social groups and activities tend to also form among clusters of same-age people. Another factor is the effect that the AIDS epidemic has had on the subculture. I have often wondered where we would be politically and socially had we not lost an entire generation of leaders, pioneers, and citizens.

One of the best antidotes to social isolation is regular participation in any activity, and going to the gym can provide the aging male with an ideal solution. It becomes a solution in two powerful ways: one, strength training will keep him strong enough to stay mobile and independent as long as possible; and two, the gym in itself and its members can be an ongoing and diverse social outlet (and one of those rare establishments in modern gay society where both young and old congregate). For Cecil Franco, the gym started out as a way to improve health, then developed into a social outlet:

> The social aspect has become more important than it was originally. The social part is powerfully reinforced by going to a gay gym and seeing all these other men who were also gay and for whatever reasons were interested in developing their bodies.
>
> In some ways, people are much more acceptable [at a gay gym]. In the beginning I felt kind of awkward, it was a new environment for me . . . but later on I realized I could actually talk with these people [he laughs]. They were much more sophisticated culturally. There were interests that we had in common—some-

> times I would run into my gay students, and then I began to realize there were older gay men who were going to the gym and I had interests in finding gay older men to socialize with. It was just nice for me to see faces of older gay men. Of course, there were the younger gay men who I found especially attractive—it was just nice to see them even though I didn't get to be conversational with them.[21]

The gym provides not just social opportunities but structure, as Cecil tells us: "Since I've retired the only structure I have is the structure I develop for myself, so the gym has become even more central than before; it's my one permanent appointment three times a week." When asked about the gym as a social outlet, Michael Meehan states: "It's becoming more important now that I'm not working because it's some place where I can see people on a regular basis, it is an important component."[22] In addition, older gay men who go to the gym on a regular basis eventually get to know the other gym goers. For example, Meehan and Franco met at the gym, and now the two old-timers often chat each other up about what's going on with their lives and with the world. As we have seen earlier, the gym provides the opportunity for many different levels and types of friendships and relationships—from the most casual to others that have the potential to evolve into significant support and social groups. Even if the extent of the socialization at the gym involves chit-chatting about retirement and the good old times between sets of exercise, this can be an important and, for some who live by themselves, possibly the only social interaction of the day.

MIDLIFE REFOCUS

An important episode in a man's life occurs when he looks inward and then outward and startlingly realizes that there is no connection between the two points of reference—this startling occurrence is better known as the *midlife crisis*. The infamous midlife crisis comes with the onset of mid-thirties or early forties, although to some of us it happens a lot sooner and to others, well, it never happens at all. Regardless of the individual circumstances, lost youth as well as lost time almost always seem to be vital to the crisis. It is probably no coincidence that this occurs invariably at the same time the body starts a transformation of its own. One of the most powerful ways that lost youth presents itself is by the lack of vigor and strength in a once energetic and sturdy body.

As gay men get older, their priorities shift dramatically. Responsibilities and demands at work increase, interpersonal relationships—whether platonic or romantic—typically become more serious and demanding, and there is a serious refocusing of energy expenditure. The high level of energy that was available during their twenties and thirties simply no longer exists. If we are lucky, we become more in tune with work, relationships, and our bodies—we clearly become more interested in not just looking fit, but feeling fit. Dinner and a movie on Saturday night and a yoga class on Sunday morning replace those late Saturday nights dancing till dawn and sleeping Sunday away. There is a lot less partying and a lot more gym. Because of the changes in priorities and the social venues that come with aging, as many gay men mature, the gym and fitness takes a more central role in their social lives.

Mind fitness becomes as important as physical fitness. As a man ages, there is a tendency to look inward for that which can center him not just physically, but mentally as well. The mind-body connection that many find today through various forms of exercise is more and more becoming the method of choice as a way to move through stages of middle age and later life.

GENERATIONAL DIFFERENCES

Visit any of the very popular resorts among older gay men in Palm Springs or Fort Lauderdale and you will find incalculable numbers of older gay men whose only bicep exercises—ever—is bringing a martini glass to their mouths. Instead of being critical, however, we need to acknowledge that older gay men simply did not have the same opportunities to work out and socialize. From civil rights (albeit limited) and nondiscrimination laws to gay pride events to gay gyms and gay television, Generations X and Y clearly have had an unmatched advantage over gay Baby Boomers and their seniors.

Historically speaking, the detonation of gay gym culture is a Generation X phenomenon. Forty years ago, exercising in general was not popular in mainstream America or any of its subcultures for that matter—except of course for the tiny segments made up of competitive athletes and bodybuilders. These were two segments which gay men in particular were not only discouraged but also generally ostracized from. When we compare the lifestyles of younger gay men with those of their older equivalents, the main differences are clearly explained in a very different set of circumstances.

When asked why more gay men his age are not involved in the gym, Lenny Simpson is quick to explain:

> One answer, obvious to me is that there are not many fifty-eight-year-olds left in urban centers like San Francisco and New York City because of the AIDS/HIV epidemic. A lot of these men, my peers, succumbed to HIV and AIDS, so our numbers are down compared with twenty- and thirty-year olds now.
>
> Some have decided to let their bodies go and pursue their minds only. A lot of these men grew up at a time when the body was not emphasized. I think as time progresses, we're going to see a lot of the guys who are in their twenties and thirties continue doing workouts until they're eighty.[23]

In the past, whether for lack of knowledge or lack of will, men chose to ignore the body, and age beset the man. In direct contrast, we are now witnessing a cultural shift in which more and more older men are taking the road less traveled. Quickly becoming one of the most significant groups of gay gym culture, the older gay male is setting an example for all of us to follow.

THE FOUNTAIN OF YOUTH

The Spanish explorer Juan Ponce De León was purportedly searching for the legendary fountain of youth when he landed in Florida in 1513. Wild voyages and explorations for the fountain have abounded in both history and mythology for centuries before and after De León, and while much has changed in the world since the time of Spanish *conquistadores,* the desire of modern men to preserve youth remains a strong and influential one.

From pomegranate juice to green tea and facials to Botox, the multibillion-dollar industry built around anti-aging and youth-preserving methods, products, and treatments is the best indication that the search for the fountain of youth not only continues but also has gained momentum. Unfortunately for you and me, the majority of such methods, products, and treatments are either out of reach or are as scientifically sound as the magic fountain.

A few exceptions provide true, though limited, preventions against the perils of aging: modern medicine, nutrition, and exercise. Of the three, exercise has proven to be the most effective method in maintaining a level of strength and energy that previously were believed to be the domain of the young. Combine the three elements, and we have a pretty good equation for maintaining health and vigor well into old age. As a fifty-three-year-old from Hawaii who took my survey wrote:

> Exercise is how one takes care of oneself. No more optional than brushing your teeth. Where else in life do you get a deal where, within limits, the more you use something the better it gets? It's just too good a deal to pass up. Exercise makes one feel good physically, emotionally, and spiritually.

Growing old presents tough challenges no doubt, and there are many things that we can do to ease the challenges. Going to the gym and getting fit is clearly not the only choice, but as Cecil told me: "my energy level is up, and I feel more a part of the world than before . . . more connected," is a good place to start.

For millennia, to age meant to decay, but in modern times the association is finally loosening. The fields of kinesiology, and more specifically exercise physiology, have established that the decay that occurs with aging is not only quite manageable but largely preventable. In addition, by maintaining a certain level of fitness as we age, we can ward off and altogether help to prevent the diseases that are killing everyone else. By being able to control the body's composition via nutrition and exercise we can manage and sometimes prevent two of the most debilitating aspects of the aging process: the loss of strength and the loss of movement. Fitness is the new fountain of youth.

Chapter 12

The Locker Room

Esteban Soto

> Just the other day, I was in the sauna, totally relaxed, feeling great after a great workout, sex being the last thing on my mind. All of a sudden, in walks this guy I've had a crush on since I joined the gym, and for the first time I see him in nothing but a towel wrapped around his beautiful and sexy athletic body. In a matter of seconds, there went my relaxation. I made an effort not to stare, but even the occasional glance was enough to give me a hard-on, and I had to casually place my hands in front of my crotch to cover my erection. At that point I couldn't get up to leave. I had no intention of acting on the urge, and I did not, but there was really nothing I could do to prevent it.[1]

All workouts begin and end in the locker room. And conversations about the gym often quickly turn to a discussion about the curious things that occur, or have the propensity to occur, between the tiled walls of the gym's wet area. More so than with any other topic discussed in this book, the locker room is a subject about which many of the gay and bisexual men I interviewed, surveyed, and talked to seemed both fascinated by yet conflicted about at the same time. It is also the one topic that brought to the table not just the most opinions but also the most divisive set of opinions—and also the one topic that some men chose not to discuss altogether.

Excitement, fear, hot, disgust, sexually charged, conflicted, ambivalent, exhilarated, trashy, shamed, and embarrassed are only some of the words that men in my research used to describe their feelings and attitudes about the locker room. How can a simple changing room elicit such a diverse set of emotional responses? Why are we fasci-

Muscle Boys: Gay Gym Culture
Published by The Haworth Press, Taylor & Francis Group, 2008.
doi:10.1300/6034_12

nated by the locker room while at the same time conflicted by it? Why do some men feel excited while others feel afraid in the locker room? Discussing these questions and examining the dynamics of the locker room is what this chapter is about.

Gay men have different attitudes about the locker room, and different feelings. As with many other things in life that make us nervous or conflicted, the diverse feelings that gay men experience toward the locker room boil down to its sexual and moral elements. Gay men perceive, experience, and feel a mixture of things toward sexual and social elements in a locker room setting. There is also a history of a well-documented correlation between the locker room and homosexuality.

THE HIGH SCHOOL LOCKER ROOM

By and large, the catalyst for the varied attitudes that gay men express toward the locker room, as well as the dynamics of the locker room, stem from their experiences as adolescents in high school locker rooms. For many of us, it was exactly in the locker room that we first experienced strong sexual urges at the sight of other boys—naked boys, to be exact. It was in the locker room where many of us—confused, excited, and afraid of these sexual urges—either battled or came to grips with our homosexuality. Let's also remember, that of course, this occurs during the years (twelve to eighteen) when most of us were not equipped to deal with the complexities of sexuality, and especially homosexuality.

Cecil, the seventy-nine-year year-old you met in Chapter 11, has vivid memories of the locker room:

> [My locker room experiences] began in junior high school, where everyone was required to take gym class. . . . I was very fearful of taking the gym class. . . . I don't think I was so much afraid of the nudity as I was afraid of actually not being up to the standards of the other boys. . . . Already in my mind I had begun fantasizing what it would be like to see the other boys naked and also fantasizing about touching them. . . . It was very difficult for me to go into the gym and to undress myself . . . because the whole act of undressing was sort of uncovering, of exposing . . . At that time, I knew I was attracted to other boys . . . and the

> clothing was a kind of a wall, that guarded us,—it guarded me from them and them from me.[2]

The high school locker room scenario is difficult for gay teens because when we are teenagers and overflowing with testosterone, we get stimulated very easily. At that age, many young men have very little control, if any at all, of when and where they get their erections. For homosexually inclined boys, those erections pop up at the sight of another naked boy in a matter of seconds. Even when not erect, the sexual urges and feelings are, for many gay boys, overpowering during those early stages of manhood.

The combination of raging hormones and sexual identity during these formative years, as Freud told us over and over, has profound outcomes in our personalities and behaviors as adults. The varied experiences—from the exciting and very good, to the very bad and terrifying—that we had in the locker room explain the varied attitudes that most of us, now as grown men, have toward the varied dynamics of the locker room.

As Cecil explains:

> It was exciting because I dearly wanted to see them naked. . . . I kind of knew that before I got to that phase in my life. . . . So that was part of it . . . and then I got focused on particular boys whom I found particularly attractive. [At this point, Cecil's face lights up with a big smile, and for a moment I can see the twelve-year-old remembering this.] There was this boy, and he was the best swimmer on the team; what I liked about him . . . it was a combination, he had this very slender, well well-shaped body, but he was also a star athlete, so he combined the beauty with the athleticism. . . . And he became a kind of role model for me . . . he became the well-defined object of attraction, who combined the physical prowess with the natural beauty.[3]

Esteban Soto shared his experience:

> When I was 16, I had my first gay experience, and during the first 60 seconds of my first sexual encounter with another man, I knew right there and then that it was right, it felt right, that there was absolutely nothing wrong with it—I knew that I was gay. Although I never had a sexual encounter in my high school

> locker room, soon after that first sexual experience the nakedness in the locker room for me was connected to my sexuality—something that I had just begun to celebrate. Although I was not particularly interested in, or good at, high school sports—and to a certain degree disliked them, going to gym class was something I looked forward to for the simple reason that I was going to be in a room full of naked boys. It was a place where I could entertain my sexuality and my sexual fantasies.[4]

But as liberal and enlightened as Esteban's adolescence was, I have known and talked to many gay men who had a very different experience from Esteban's and battled those same urges for years, some of them for more than twenty years and longer. For them the locker room was a place of frustration, of shame, and of fear. It was a place where those feelings they were trying to suppress invariably—and, to make matters worse, sometimes literally—came up.

Although Cecil Franco can recall some very pleasant memories, especially when he thinks of the "swimmer," he also has other memories that were not as good:

> It was terrifying because of this fear of exposure and also the norms of my family where you know, you don't undress in front of other people. Nudity at our home, was something that was strictly forbidden, so we were not allowed to run around the house naked . . . probably because I have three sisters, and they were always scurrying in and out of the bathroom.

The mixture of feelings that gay men have toward the locker room very often has more to do with what the locker room was there for: gym class. As I discussed in Chapter 8, high school athletics are troublesome, to say the least, for many gay men.

The visuals alone in the locker room are capable of triggering in many gay men the most exciting memories as well as the most painful ones. Something as simple as a row of lockers, group showers, or a naked body standing in front of the lockers can remind some of us of a jock we had a crush on in high school, bringing to memory those incomparable feelings of lust and excitement some of us felt. But the same naked body standing in front of those lockers, for someone else, can bring to mind a very different memory: not fitting in athletically, or worse. Gay youth are still experiencing that one kid who taunted or terrorized him or even physically attacked him while in the locker room. That unfortunate experience brings up the painful feelings of shame, fear, and helplessness that accompany verbal or physical attacks. To complicate matters even more, many gay men will vacillate between both scenarios in their memory repertoire, sometimes simultaneously.

THE MORAL DILEMMA: SEX IN PUBLIC PLACES

The locker room and sexual dynamics present in it become a controversial topic. Social etiquette dictates that sex in public spaces is not appropriate unless those public spaces have been designated as such, as in the case of sex clubs or bathhouses. Even these designated sexual public spaces are so controversial that they are often debated, protested, and shut down. Sex in public spaces represents a social and moral dilemma problem that has been debated since the times of Dionysus to current arguments debating the place of gay bathhouses in modern urban centers. In my research, sex in the locker room proved to be one of the most debated topics when it comes to gay gym culture, second only to steroids. A great deal of men who participated in my research wanted to talk about sex and the potential for sex in the locker room—in many cases it was the only topic that some of them were interested in discussing in-depth at all. Almost immediately after only the first few interviews and surveys, I realized that the number one reason why people wanted to discuss this subject so much is because I was approaching them with an academic and honestly nonjudgmental interest in the subject, which is typically not the case. I offered them a safe space to discuss the matter, safe from political correctness, safe from having to be morally correct, and safe from judgments. Once we got the giggles and smirks out of the way they were able to tell me how they really felt. They also often told me that it was the first time they had discussed and entertained the subject so honestly.

In surveys and interviews I asked the question: "How do you feel about men who engage in or look for sex in the locker room?" Surprisingly, 43 percent (2,053) of respondents answered, "It's a personal decision" (see Figure 12.1). I found it surprising because when I conducted the initial and much smaller survey in San Francisco, I figured that the response came largely from a very socially liberal city where, if for nothing else, people here would choose the "it's a per-

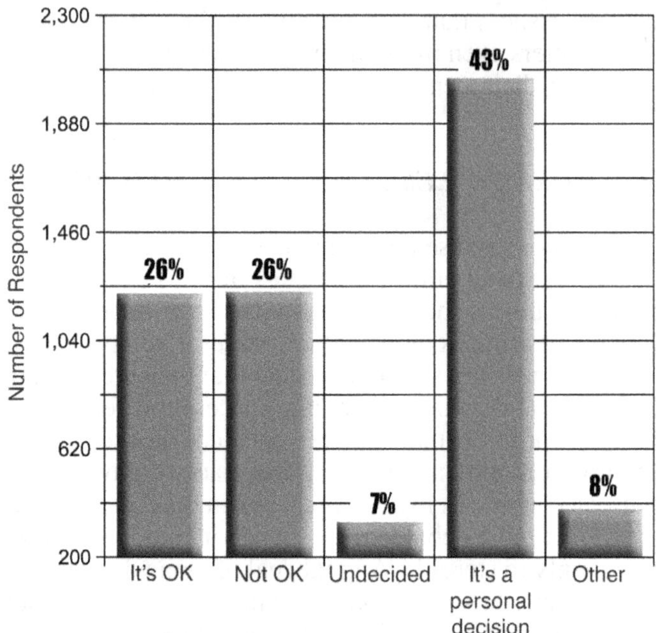

FIGURE 12.1. Different perspectives regarding sex in the locker room.

sonal decision" answer because in liberal San Francisco it would be the open-minded and politically correct thing to say. But I was wrong. In fact, when compared with the larger survey that included several thousand gay and bisexual (and a small percentage of straight) men from across the nation and around the world, including well-known sexually conservative havens such as the Midwest, the South, and even the Middle East, there was very little if any difference.

The other 57 percent of respondents were split between answering that the behavior is "It's OK" (26 percent or 1,219) and "Not OK" (26 percent or 1,228); a smaller group (7 percent or 334) were "undecided." Survey respondents were also given the option to write in their own specific answers to the question rather than select one from the multiple choices given; 8 percent of respondents chose this route, and they had plenty to say. A few people chastised me for the words I chose to use in the question, telling me that "engage in" and "look for" sex are two different actions. While they have a point, it also became very clear to me that most people who answered the question either approved or disapproved regardless of whether one is "looking for" or "engaging in" sex. The 386 different opinions skewed heavily in either one direction or the other—or literally between "it's hot" and "it's disgusting," with one exemption, the many who stated that their answers would change depending on whether the gym was straight or gay, or "It depends on the gym. A straight gym—no. A gay gym—maybe."

To some extent the argument that fuels the controversies of sex in public spaces comes down to the differences in sexual attitudes between men and women and how these differences determine and define social decorum. Most women would not only be disinterested, but appalled, at the idea of a quick sexual encounter with a total stranger following their lunchtime workout, while many men—gay and straight—on the other hand are not only willing, but willing to go the extra mile to find one.

Sex in public spaces often boils down to a battle between our natural sexual urges and social protocol dictating to what extent we ought to act—or not act—on them, and how. Furthermore, historically, for gay men, this conflict of nature versus nurture in regard to sexual behavior is something that extends well into many other areas of our lives. To a great extent, coming out and accepting our homosexuality, for many of us, has been a rejection of mainstream moral beliefs about what is right and what is wrong. Historically, society has not only disapproved of sex between men in the locker room, or any public space for that matter, it has disapproved of sex between men altogether—everywhere and anywhere. Let's not forget that it has only been a few years (2003) since sodomy was officially decriminalized in the United States;[5] and prior to this very recent date, gay men were thrown in jail for having sex—not just in public, but in the privacy of their bedrooms. Anti-sodomy laws still exist in several other nations.

Because our feelings about sex in public will often correspond to how we feel about homosexuality in general, there is an understandable tendency for some gay men to feel about sex in public as unapologetically or as shameful about it as they might feel about their sexuality in general. Yet, historically sex between men in public spaces of the locker room variety is as well documented as the controversies that the topic generates.

I have many times encountered disapproving attitudes, including many gay men, who criticize the gay facilities because of the sex that occurs in the locker rooms. What these people fail miserably to recognize is that locker room sex between men is not a gay gym phenomenon: locker room sex has been occurring for millennia, before the first gay gym ever opened. Locker room sex is a phenomenon of opportunity—simple laws of supply and demand.

If we go back to the first-ever gymnasium, the ancient Greek gymnasia, we find very interesting parallels to today's locker room dynamics. In fact, the ancient gymnasiums were much more elaborate in terms of wet areas, changing rooms, and grooming practices, than most modern gyms. For one, at the entrance of the gymnasiums the first room was the *apodyterion,* or undressing room, where you were required to disrobe completely. Second, the ancient Greek gym goers bathed both before and after every workout, and in the literature we can find references to lavish baths and Jacuzzi-like hot tubs. Third, the baths were followed by a visit to the "oil room" where the athletes would oil and powder their naked bodies before wrestling or working out. Fourth, it was commonplace for the athletes to massage each other—in the nude—following their workouts. Though the Greeks did not have saunas or steam rooms, there is no doubt that the wet areas of the ancient gymnasiums got pretty damn hot.

Although the ancient Greek gymnasiums were places where men would meet male sexual partners, there are no direct references to sex occurring right there and then. However, given the nature of men as well as the nature of the highly charged sexual energy of the Greek gymnasiums, where statues of Eros presided and where men interested in having sex with men were naked not only in the changing rooms, but everywhere in the gym, I am quite confident that it did.

Following the Greek era, the past 2,000 years are peppered with a rich history of bathhouses (i.e., Turkish baths, saunas, etc.). The bathhouse might now be a space that gay men have preserved as public sex havens but for millennia they were public bathing places. Most rational historians do not argue that these bathhouses presented the opportunity and space for a sexual encounter between two or more men. In fact, how the gay bathhouse came to be as a gay institution was organically—as historians have told us repeatedly, public bathhouses were public sex spaces for men way before the first *official* gay bathhouse ever opened.

In more recent history, as far as gyms go, sex between men in the locker room started to occur as soon as the first modern gyms opened. For several decades before the onset of gay liberation, the YMCA's locker rooms in the cities of New York and San Francisco were notorious during the first half of the last century as places not just where men could find male sex partners but as places where they could have sex.

What we find in 2,500 years of documented history is a clear and unarguable historical connection between locker rooms and sex between men.

THE VOYEUR AND THE EXHIBITIONIST

> To hook up in the locker room was always something I wanted to do, but could never do it, because my boyfriend was always with me at the gym. Finally I got the chance, and I was totally addicted. I would spend all day thinking about going there; I would spend my whole day thinking, "I can't wait to go to the gym tonight and hook up . . ." And my workouts became a total chore, because I wanted to go straight to the locker room. I'd force myself to work out, but I would definitely cut the workout short because I wanted to get in the locker room. [6]

Most of the sexual dynamics in the locker room fall into two categories: voyeurism and exhibitionism.

The majority of men who walk into a locker room tend to fall into the voyeur category—he who watches. The voyeur experience can be as casual and brief as walking through the locker room to wash your hands or put your gym bag in a locker while very casually observing those who are naked and/or changing or as involved as masturbating across the shower from another naked body or watching two of your gym peers exchange blow jobs in the steam room while they are sitting next to you.

A smaller percentage of men fall into the exhibitionist category. Often the voyeur and the exhibitionist are the same person, but not always. From my observations, it is more likely for an exhibitionist to be a voyeur than for a voyeur to also be an exhibitionist. And I presume that this is because simply watching is a lot easier and less risky than performing. Besides, whether one walks in the locker room with voyeuristic intentions or not, sometimes it just happens for the simple reason that we humans are curious animals; we stop and look when something out of the ordinary occurs in our environment.

The exhibitionist in the locker room is also a master at the art of doing nothing, except that he does so while in the nude or mostly nude. At times, he does so in the steam room or the sauna, where doing nothing is the point. The exhibitionist is not just relaxing, taking in the steam, but is instead letting the steam out. At other times, he is more active and moves from the showers to the steam room to the sauna, over and over again.

Jason explains to me his locker room routine:

> I would undress, put on a towel, start in the dry sauna, see what was going on, then go back and forth between the dry sauna and the wet sauna. There was almost always something going on, but I couldn't wait to get in there. I'd try to relax, but it would be hard because I'm so excited, I'm waiting for someone to come in. Sometimes it would get to the point where it would get too hot in there for me and then I'd keep saying, "OK, I'll wait five more minutes, maybe someone will show up" . . . and someone would finally show up and something would start to happen but I'd have to leave 'cause I felt like I was going to have a heart attack. It was already too hot, and I'm nervous that I'm going to get caught. It's just nerve-wracking altogether.

A few days after discussing this topic with Tom Madonna, whom you met in Chapter 6, Tom came to me and told me how after paying attention during those last few days, he noticed how some gym members have in fact "mastered the art of doing nothing," in order to hang out in the locker room. He then described a scenario that many of us who go to the gym regularly can recognize:

> I've seen guys with a pumice stone, doing their feet, and doing their nails, and men with travel kits; they'll shave, condition their hair, and spend all this time in front of the mirror doing their treatments. And during this time they'll have one eye on the mirror and one eye on the steam room door, and what they'll do is put their stuff down at the opportunity of someone going in

> the steam room. They can spend a lot of time in the locker room looking busy, like they have a purpose, but they are just waiting for something to come up in the steam room. Because there's only so much 100-degree steam you can take before you pass out.
>
> There are people who do this once in a while, but then there are the professionals—they're very aggressive. They are so brazen and bold, they throw down the shaving cream and race into the steam room and drop their towel and try to get it on.[7]

A straight male friend of mine who has noticed this dynamic has come up with the term "shower monkeys" to describe the men who for no defined purpose spend a lot of time "hanging around the showers."

Highly sexual environments are so common at some popular gyms in San Francisco, New York City, and Los Angeles (among many other cities) that jumping in the steam room after a shower (and during peak hours) almost always opens up the doors for a sexual encounter to occur or at the very least, to witness. Interestingly enough, and contrary to common opinion, we often find these highly sexual environments more common at "straight" gyms versus those that are primarily gay. This occurs for two reasons. One, a heavier "straight" male clientele brings to the showers a lot of men who find in the locker room one of the very few places, if not the only one, where they can sexually interact with other men. And two, some of these gyms simply provide more spaces, such as steam rooms and saunas, where sexual encounters can actually occur. Many new gyms, in cities and towns big and small, are starting to design locker rooms without steam rooms (because of the steam you can't seen what's going on) and positioning the sauna (if they put one in) with big glass doors in plain view of the doorway. They are doing this to discourage the locker room from being used as a sex club by its male members.

Exhibitionism and Body Image

A true exhibitionist does not simply feel comfortable being naked in front of others, he enjoys it, and to various degrees gets off on it. In gay gym culture we can find common physical traits among men who like to show off. These traits are best described in terms of size—big muscles and big penises. Locker room exhibitionists desire to draw attention to their bodies and sometimes the genitals, which in turn feeds their ego in one way or another. Although our focus here is specific to males, I am told that female exhibitionists in the ladies locker room are also common. Furthermore, while quite often the exhibitionist has sex on his mind, it's not always the case; sometimes it is purely a sexless ego feed. Exhibitionism has no simple definition because its occurrence is influenced to different degrees and by diverse factors, which are complicated amongst themselves—from true narcissism to complex psychological issues to just trying to get laid. As Jason told me, he "works out hard in the weight room" so that he will "look good in the steam room."

Some men, like Jason, feel comfortable being naked in the locker room only when they feel confident about the way their bodies look. As Jason tells me, as much as he loved the locker room:

> I didn't really want to go in there unless I was pumped up. I would work out for an hour, but specifically working out body parts that would look bigger so that when I got in the locker room I would look better.

I have noticed a few men who shower and walk around naked only while on a cycle of steroids; between cycles they do not even change in the locker room.

Another group of men, regardless of musculature, clearly enjoy the attention garnered toward another body part—their penis. Quite often, the guys who feel the most comfortable walking around the locker room naked are those who are very well hung; they clearly enjoy the double takes. I had a friend confide in me that he doesn't shower at the gym because he thinks his dick is too small. We men do a lot of comparing in the locker room. This is a competitive and curiosity element that occurs regardless of sexual preference or sexual interest—even straight men still size up the other guys and their packages, more often than not in comparison with themselves.

Lastly, there is another component that completely changes the dialogue of exhibitionism and body image in the locker room (and outside of it as well): cultural and ethnic upbringings and their associated social norms. For example, many Europeans or Brazilians think nothing about being naked and walking around naked in a locker room—it is a nonissue. On the other hand, Americans and those influenced by cultures from most Middle Eastern, and quite a few of the Asian and Latin American countries *do think about it*—a lot—sometimes more than would seem healthy or even practical. Varying attitudes about nudity in different cultures have been written about quite a bit and are nothing new. But I have to admit that when I actually set out to pay close attention to the different ways men carry themselves when they are undressing or getting dressed in the locker room the differences in comfort level are truly often so dramatic that it was both informative and sometimes painful to watch.

On one side of this coin is the archetypal European man who grew up going to nude beaches with the family on holidays, where being nude was what everyone did and nudity was simply normal. This guy can undress in the locker room with the same comfort level that everyone does at home every day, and does not even find it necessary to wrap a towel around his waist as he walks from the lockers to the showers. He also acknowledges his environment and those in it in the same way that office workers are expected to acknowledge their office and coworkers. When he's nude his personality does not change: he'll make eye contact, chat, and even stop to greet a friend or acquaintance and engage in a conversation. On the flip side is the characteristic American guy who grew up influenced by a culture that although is oversaturated with sex talk and nude imagery, cannot divorce itself from the association that both have as dirty and shameful. And this is where it gets interesting, not to mention noticeable. What is most noticeable is the change in personality and body language that many guys exhibit just by walking in the door of the changing room, by switching into an almost immediate level of discomfort that is most noticeable by a self-imposed effort to avoid eye contact as well as casual social interaction, even by the most outgoing guys. These are the types of guys who can spot you across the gym and even greet you from that far away, but don't even "see" or "notice" you in the locker room even if you're standing only three feet away. There is an unwritten moral code that says that naked guys have no business talking to or even worse, looking at each other.

In the locker room the seriousness of discomfort can also be observed in other common behavior patterns. For example, many guys will not even change their shirts while other guys are in the locker room, and others go as far as going into one of the toilet stalls to change; others will keep their towel wrapped around their waist even as they put on their underwear; and on the far end of the spectrum we find others that take extreme and impractical measures in order to stay covered by actually showering with their underwear on.

Cultural differences when it comes to nudity confuse the subject of exhibitionism because a lot of times exhibitionism is defined by cultural perceptions of what is acceptable in terms of nakedness, even if the nakedness has absolutely no ulterior motive. Of course the different behaviors toward nudity are not only influenced by cultural norm, and might be defined by psychological variances, but they almost always correlate with one's upbringing. Because of this, it is difficult to truly measure exhibitionism or what may be perceived as such. Is the guy walking around the locker room naked being an exhibitionist or is he just comfortable being naked in public? We don't really know, do we? Truth is, it could be either.

LOCKER ROOM SEX

Given that locker rooms are not intended sexual spaces, it is this watching-and-being-watched dynamic that constitutes the sexual acts that predominate locker room sexuality. In both cases, either the voyeur or the exhibitionist is safe to act out on his sexuality without making physical contact with another person or involving man-on-man sex, thereby staying within the range of what is allowed. While actual contact (touching, oral, or anal) sex is not allowed in gymnasium locker rooms, there are no written rules about looking. For many men, this is perfectly fine; they get off on just watching and/or being watched.

The most common sex act in the locker room is masturbation: typically, one man will begin masturbating in the sauna or the steam room while another man is present. At this point if there is mutual interest, the second man will also start masturbating, and often the two men engage in mutual masturbation. Masturbation is on some occasions followed by oral sex, and on rare occasions anal sex. The same scenario often involves more than one man, and at times several, turning the situation into group sex.

> [In the locker room] I never had penetration sex. It was always just jerking off, which was most of the time, or oral—pretty much it would be like a big circle jerk. [When it was oral] it was them giving me oral, I never sucked anyone off. I would have, but they always beat me to it.[8]

Given that sex in the locker room is considered taboo, it's interesting to note that nearly half of men have participated in it. In my survey I posed the question, "Have you ever engaged in any type of sexual activity while in the locker room of any gym?" and 41 percent (1,955) of total survey respondents said "Yes." Although that represents a huge percentage, a slight majority, 57 percent (2,749) of respondents answered, "No." Lastly, 2 percent (76) of respondents did not feel comfortable answering the question and opted for the "Prefer not to answer" choice (which as any Freudian will tell you in most cases means yes) (see Figure 12.2).

An interesting question to ask at this point is, just what is the line between looking and touching? This, of course, is a loaded question, pun intended. Although some men, like Jason, will plan in advance and actively look for a sexual encounter in the locker room, many others just happen to be at the right place at the right time (or wrong place at the right time). A sexual encounter is facilitated in the locker room for two simple reasons: the involved parties are naked, and men get sexually stimulated quite easily. Men who are homosexually in-

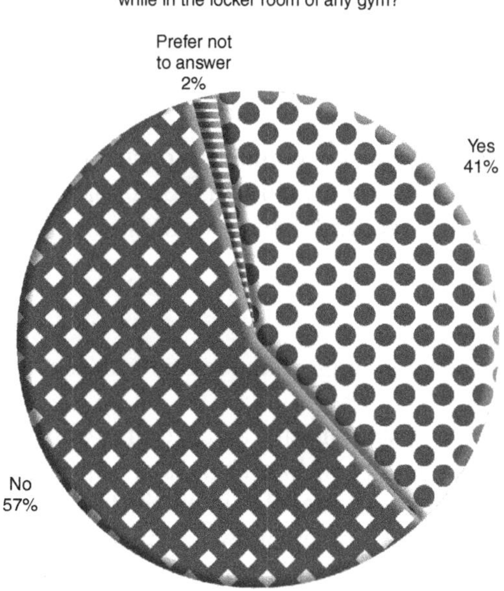

FIGURE 12.2. Percentage of men who have engaged in locker room sex.

clined at any level will be visually stimulated at the sight of other naked men. Since talking in showers, steam rooms, and saunas is not common between strangers (and sometimes discouraged as they are places intended for quiet time), body language becomes the means for an invitation or acceptance of actual sex. Something as simple as making eye contact, a suggestive gaze, or touching of one's body can send a message of sexual interest to the other party. The interest is at times displayed and responded to with an erection. Once an erection is present, there is no question as to the possibilities that can lead to actual sex. So, the line between looking and touching is, more often than not, drawn by your penis, and more specifically its angle. The correlation is, simply put, a linear one.

Surprisingly enough, some of the heterosexual male respondents to my survey responded that they thought it was "OK" or "it's a personal decision" for men to engage in or look for sex in the locker room. Though most of them also stated that it was OK as long as they were not actively pursued for it or as long as they did not have to see it, several of them understand why it occurs. As one of them told me, "I understand why it happens; I know that if I was taking a shower and there was a naked woman in the shower across from me, I would get excited as well." Another straight male respondent went so far as to tell me he was envious of gay guys: "You guys have it made," he said, pointing out how much more difficult if not impossible it is for a casual male-female sexual encounter to occur on the gym premises. The reality is that if straight men had the opportunity for casual sex with women in the locker room many would not hesitate to act on it.

The Actors

Who are the men who engage in locker room sex, and why do they do it?

Damon Xiang (a pseudonym), a successful, thirty-something accountant and bodybuilder in San Francisco who is partnered to another white-collar professional also in his thirties, told me that he and his partner have decided on a somewhat open relationship in which they both feel that the anonymity of sexual encounters in the locker room is the type of sex that is allowed outside the relationship—"unthreatening to the relationship" as well as an "exciting" escapade.[9]

Jason Six, who has shared with me his most intimate accounts about his locker room sexual encounters (including graphic details that I have not published, this being a serious discussion undistracted by erotica) told me that although he is thrilled by the occurrences he does not talk about them with his partner, as such encounters are not allowed. Putting aside moral judgments on monogamy and fidelity, in this case, locker room sex allows Jason to get away with unacceptable, outside-the-relationship, sexual encounters with minimal risk of being caught. Although Jason would like to share the experiences with his partner, he knows that his partner would not react positively. In fact, he tells me:

> My new boyfriend would never allow it. He is the type who would say, as far as what goes on in the locker room, that it is improper and disgusting. He is a prude to say the least. He'll say things like, "If I ever see it, I'll turn those people in."

Though for Jason's relationship the locker room flings pose a threat, for other coupled gay men the sexual escapades are just fine. As a forty-one-year-old from Indiana, wrote:

> I belong to a couple of gyms. One is a gay club. I engage in sex as much as twice per week and have sex with about 100 men per year. As I get in better shape, I am much more selective—hence less sex. I have a partner of eight years who is cool with all of this.

Of course, not all men who engage in or look for sex in the locker room are partnered. In fact, many do so precisely because they are not. For this other group of men, locker room sex offers a quick fix to an ongoing need. The easy solution appeals to a lot of men who are sexually starved, without having to deal with the trials and tribulations of dating or investing the time into looking for sex partners through other more time-consuming venues.

STRAIGHT MEN WHO HAVE SEX WITH MEN

Some guys feel comfortable enough to admit and even share their locker room "very hot" stories, but many others will not. This is especially the case when these guys also happen to be "straight." Less talked about, and a lot less in your face, is the fact that some straight men use the steam room to experience more than steam. Nine percent (9 percent) of my survey respondents (496 men) identified as "bisexual" (some are married and have girlfriends). Another 1 percent of survey respondents (51 men) identified solely as "straight," and 1.2 percent identified as "questioning (68 men). From the latter two groups of 119 straight and questioning men, as well as with a few other straight men I interviewed who admitted to same-sex encounters in the locker room, the fact that "straight" men partake in locker room sex with other men is more than palpable. Surprisingly, some of them feel more comfortable having sex with another man in the locker room than many of the gay men I interviewed. Not surprisingly they partake for the same reasons that gay men do: because it's "available," "anonymous," and "hot." Some straight-identified men seek out and prefer encounters with other straight-identified men as opposed to encounters with gay-identified men, mainly in an effort to ensure anonymity.

> There were of course many men there for sex with other men but I would say only a minority of them thought of themselves as gay. Many had girlfriends or wives. I liked these guys best as I thought they would be less risky if encountered outside the locker room situation . . . i.e., they had to be straight-acting and not out so as not to expose me in public. (Anonymous interviewee)

This same man was very open and relaxed, even excited to discuss with me his many locker room romps over a period of ten years; he was actually more concerned with how discussing the subject for this book might bring awareness to the nonmembers of the club:

> I don't know who your target readership might be but it sort of concerns me a bit that your book might make straight guys aware of stuff in locker rooms that they are oblivious to now. Not great for guys like me who presently use such places to hook up with other like-minded guys.

Many gays who disapprove of locker room sexual encounters oppose them precisely because they feel that men who have sex in the locker room "give gay culture a bad name," because they *assume* that all shower monkeys are gay. They are wrong. The truth is that the men who are giving each other blowjobs at your neighborhood gym may or may not be citizens of gay culture; in fact many will tell you flat out that they are straight. And to an extent they are; they are your straight male neighbors, the guys who are married, have girlfriends, and children and for whatever reason identify as straight—except in the sauna. My point here is not to criticize or try and analyze the sexuality of these "straight" men who engage in locker room sex with other men, especially within the very limited definitions of labels such as "gay" and "straight." Rather, if we are going to use these labels and be concerned with the reputation that gay culture has in the mainstream when it comes to men having sex with one another in the locker room, it is not only gay men who do participate but straight men as well. The truth of the matter is that "gay" men in many, many cases would be unable to "give gay culture a bad name," if it was not with a little help from the "straight" guy who was sucking his dick in the steam room. As another of these straight married men admitted to me when I asked him if he related in any way or form to gay culture:

> I love sex with men once in a while, but I'm predominantly straight. I'm married. Why would I identify with an entire culture over something I do just a few times a year? That would be like moving to Italy because I like to eat pasta once in a while. (Anonymous interviewee)

A straight-identified male who is curious or simply enjoys gay sex can engage in a sexual encounter with another male in a locker room without having to walk into a gay-identified establishment such as a bar, a gay sex club, or a bathhouse. For a lot of these men who do not want to, or cannot, identify as gay it is not always an easy thing or a reasonable option to "go to a bathhouse," or "take it home," as many gay survey respondents suggested. For example, in San Francisco every Friday night hundreds of (mostly gay) guys have absolutely no problem standing outside in a line of circuit boys, leather men, club kids, and drag queens (as hundreds of cars drive by) to get into Fag Fridays (a popular gay nightclub in San Francisco), or to go into Blow Buddies (a sex club) on the same block. Yet, the same Friday night routine (under most circumstances) would be terrifying for a straight-identified male who is curious about gay sex. In fact many straight men have sex in the locker room with other men because it is their only outlet to same-sex sexual encounters.

In summary, there is not one answer when we ask who are the men who engage in locker room sex. *Why* they do it is a little easier to answer. The simplest one of course is based on the laws of supply and demand: the sex is available to men who want it. Men, both gay and straight, simply get sexually worked up and partake *because they can*. Aside from this, there are two undercurrent and recurring factors that we find common in these locker room sexual encounters: the thrill and the anonymity.

When I ask Jason why the locker room sex was so exciting to him even though it was also nerve-wracking, he tells me:

> Because it was anonymous; I knew that it was going to be with someone relatively hot since I'm at the gym and everybody there is somewhat good looking. [He works out at a very popular gym in West Hollywood.] I knew it was going to be on totally neutral ground—you know, sex in the locker room never leaves the locker room. There are guys at the gym who I've hooked up with who I couldn't even tell you who they were. Once you're done, for me anyway, it's like it never happened, totally no strings attached—and that is what I liked about it.[10]

The danger of getting caught and rebelling against social norms adds, for many other men, a layer of excitement that is absent from the sex they can have in the comfort of their own homes. As one sixty-year-old from Florida, who took my survey wrote:

> I have had sex in the locker room of my gym, but my partner at the time was in fact my "partner/lover." He just liked the exhibitionist aspect of public sex. So the incidents were rare, but did occur. Generally, I am not in the gym for cruising or for sex. And generally I am annoyed by people who are obviously there for reasons other than working out.

Many of the people who disapprove of sex in the locker room were quick to tell me that those men who engage in it, should "take it home" or "get a room." As reasonable as those answers might seem to many of us they can also prove narrow-minded; what I have learned in my research is that "taking it home," or "getting a room," would ruin the locker room experience for those who thrill on it. For many men, the appeal of a sexual encounter in the locker room lies in its anonymity, even if they were in a position to take it somewhere else, the encounter would disengage from the sexual fantasy and lose its appeal. Unfortunately, an easy answer does not always solve a complicated topic.

THE BASHFUL

This brings us to the other side of the coin: the men who do not participate in the locker room aerobics. This group is made up of two categories: those men who will not engage in sex in the locker room so as not to violate social etiquette, and those who would like to but are simply too shy.

For these men, the matter is one of social approval versus one of sexual gratification. The larger attitude here is that sex in the locker room is not socially or morally accepted and that like other social norms and mores this is one that we should observe without further discussion. Interestingly enough, many of those who admitted to having had a sexual encounter at one point or another still feel that is it "not OK" to engage in sexual encounters or to even look for sex in the locker room. And many of these men will shower at home to avoid the situation.

When asked if he showers at the gym, a forty-six-year-old resported that he showers at the gym only "sometimes," because there is "too much sexual energy sometimes—hard to resist." And although he has engaged in locker room sex, he still feels that it is "not OK," "myself included."

Many of those who reported not showering at the gym at all said that they do not because: "It feels too cruisy to shower at the gym," responded a thirty-seven-year-old. . . . Another thirty-seven-year-old said that he avoids the locker room showers because he is "not into sex at the gym, that is the dark side of gay gyms."

A thirty-two-year-old who works out four to five times a week responded: "fantasy-wise, it's hot, but in reality there is a time and place for everything." He then adds:

> Cruising is much different than sex. I cruise, and it's fun to be cruised to a point. There are certain public arenas that I do not

> feel having sex is appropriate, mainly and mostly public bathrooms and locker rooms. Fantasizing and role-playing about it can be very hot . . . that is what sex clubs and Steamworks [a bathhouse in Berkeley, California] are for.

The second category includes another group of men who are simply shy or self-conscious. Many voyeurs fall into this category: they will watch but never participate. Self-consciousness about body image plays a big role here; some of these men would actually want to participate and often fantasize about it, but they do not even feel comfortable undressing in front of others. The reason for being reserved are as varied as they come—from feeling too skinny or too fat to having insecurities about penis size and at other times cultural and religious influences.

Body image has a lot to do with some of the more reserved gym members. A forty-one-year-old who has been working out for twenty-three years responded that "I had a major body image problem fifteen years ago that changes in diet and workout regime and attitude have helped." Although he now describes his body as athletic and told me that he is satisfied with the way he looks, he also responded that: "I don't like to be seen naked in public. I don't like being looked over and/or checked out."

Another man summed it up: "look and talk, but don't touch!" And another who admits having had sexual encounters in the locker room states that it is not OK because it's "not generally a good idea to be too indiscreet."

From religious upbringings and conservative values to penis envy and penis-size insecurity, the men who disapprove of locker room sex do so for many different and complicated reasons. I had this conversation with a well-known former porn star and was surprised to find that outside of film sets, he is too shy to even change in the locker room, let alone get naked and hop in the shower in front of others. So, attitudes about locker room sex are a personal issue that on some occasions have a lot more to do with how someone feels, their upbringing, and belief system than with how they look. Likewise, throughout the years, I have observed many people for whom attitudes about sexual encounters in the locker room have nothing to do with social etiquette and everything to do with a reflection of themselves and more specifically body image.

Surprisingly, a lot of the men who have never engaged in locker room sex feel that it is okay for others to do it. The responses included: "As long as they are respectful of people who don't want to participate," "As long as it doesn't create an uncomfortable atmosphere," and "As long as it doesn't violate my personal space."

Other gay men just find the whole locker room dynamics too damn distracting. One man in his mid-forties recently told me that he actually liked the locker room too much. He in fact liked the locker room so much so that it became way too distracting from his workouts. He used to have sex in the locker room all the time and spent a lot of time in there, but nowadays he prefers to change at home and will not shower at the gym in an effort to avoid being distracted from his workouts.

GEOGRAPHICAL AND ENVIRONMENTAL DIFFERENCES

Adding to the complexity of the locker room argument is that not all locker rooms are created equal and for a fair and balanced argument we must factor in a few geographical and environmental differences.

For example, some of my survey respondents who live in rural American and European areas have never been exposed to, or even witnessed, let alone participated in, sexual locker room encounters. Their gyms are very basic, and the locker room is simply a bathroom or just a changing room with none or very limited wet areas, so sexual encounters are virtually impossible. Some of these respondents wrote to me and told me that locker room sex is something that they have only read about. One respondent in rural England wrote and told me that he had actually questioned if locker room sex was nothing other than an urban myth.

Other survey participants have access to more modern facilities, but live in extremely conservative areas where the locker rooms are extremely sterile of social interaction and where even a glance at another guy carries the potential of getting your ass kicked instead of laid. Yet another group live in areas where gyms are family oriented, resulting in children being in the locker room, which completely changes the dialogue. It's one thing to walk in the locker room and notice a "daddy I'd like to fuck," and another when's he's got the kids with him and a bag of diapers.

We also find huge differences in locker room dynamics and demographics even in urban areas where locker room sex is common. The most significant difference is the demographic of the participants—those who partake and those who do not and the facilities themselves. For example, when visiting family in Saint Petersburg, Florida, I worked out at a large, chain, popular gym. At this gym, where the membership is primarily straight and middle aged, there was plenty of locker room action going on, but the participants were for the most part older men, many of them of retirement age. To find young men cruising the wet areas at this particular gym is not utterly impossible, but it is rare.

At other times, I would jump in the car and drive across the bay to Tampa where I would work out at another gym owned by the same chain. At this other gym, the membership base is also primarily straight, more urban and also younger, ranging from college age to guys in their forties. Yet, there was so much cruising and action going on that I felt as if I was back in a gay San Francisco gym. Interestingly enough, this is considered one of the "straight" gyms in Tampa. Across town, there are two popular gyms among gay men, where the membership base is about 50 percent straight and 50 percent gay. Yet neither of the two gyms rank high in terms of locker room cruising, let alone sex. What's the difference? Neither of the two heavily gay populated gyms have a steam room, whereas the straight gym does.

When it comes to sex in the locker room gay men hold an unbreakable double standard defined not just by opportunity but also by physical attraction. Furthermore, many men who have strong opinions about sexual encounters in the locker room are basing their opinions on limited experience and exposure at their particular gyms. What I learned in my research is that quite often, it is the age and looks of those who cruise the locker room that will determine other people's participation as well as the opinions and feelings regarding the behavior. Generally speaking, many of the men who disapprove of locker room cruising are the younger guys who dislike the older men cruising them. But the same younger guys will take a completely different stance toward the younger guys they consider more attractive.

The following statement from a twenty-seven-year-old from Connecticut mirrors a very predominant sentiment expressed to me hundreds of times by younger survey and interview respondents:

> I guess I don't care about cruising as long as people do it discreetly and try to stay within their league. What I don't like are the men who are rather out-of-shape and much older and who constantly leer and cruise the younger guys. I've had to ask a guy to stop hovering when I was trying to change. I've had guys be extremely obvious—follow me around, go to the shower, etc. It's just silly. What's weird is when older guys get offended that I'm not interested, because they never seem interested in each other, but rather only the younger guys.

A twenty-five-year-old construction worker in Texas wrote, "Depends on the situation, it's not fun to be cruised by someone you're not attracted to, if it's mutual then it's hot."

Older men bestowing unwanted advances on the younger ones in the locker room, creating an uncomfortable situation, is a conflict that I discussed at length during many of my interviews. The gym is one of those very few places where older and younger members of our community congregate, and uncomfortable situations between the two groups are bound to happen. For any subculture or community, this is a problem. Although the situation does occur among men of the same age, most people agree (and I have observed this to be true) that it is more common between older and younger men. It is not always the advance in itself that it is unwanted, but that it is excessive. But in all fairness, this is not always the case, and many young men will overreact to a casual advance as if they had been severely insulted or physically violated, a reaction they don't have toward those of the same age or the men they might find attractive under the same circumstances.

I can understand both sides of the equation. On one hand, I have myself experienced the unwanted advances, sometimes by men who are relentless and will not take no for an answer. On the other hand, the attraction that leads to a sexual advance is a natural reaction; whether in the locker room or on the street I do not think that anyone should limit their behavior to conform to ideals supporting ageism. Besides, in my research I found that many younger men welcome and enjoy the advances from the older ones.

Out of the discussions I had with both young and older men in regard to this scenario, two suggestions kept coming: base behavior and actions with moderation and respect. That is, pay attention as to whether an advance would be welcomed or unwarranted; and more important, respect someone's decision and space once an indication of rejection has been given.

BOYS WILL BE BOYS

Whether our own experiences in the high school locker room are good or bad, one is thing is clear: those experiences have a profound and sometimes life-lasting effect on us as young males. The serious implications of such experiences in high school or even college athletics are something that gets lost today in cheap triviality. Many of us—approvingly or disapprovingly—joke and discuss the sexual dynamics of the locker room as simply as right or wrong; meanwhile, we ignore the stratum of complex possibilities behind the different behaviors.

Whether one is candidly cruising or being bashful, an exhibitionist or a voyeur, what is clear is the level of conflict that we find between the different attitudes toward sex in the locker room. The men who approve of it find it thrilling and exiting; the ones who disapprove find it unbecoming and at times offensive. To complicate matters more, a great deal of men I talked to are split between the two—between approval and disapproval, between wanting to participate in locker room sex and condemning it, between doing it and then feeling guilty or ashamed about it. Often what creates the conflict is that a sexual situation finds us completely unprepared—as Esteban told us at the beginning of this chapter.

A lot of men will be insulted and offended if they are approached or pursued in the locker room by someone they find unattractive, but the attitude changes almost completely when the opportunity arises with someone they find attractive. Even if they find it unbecoming or improper to act on it, as Esteban did, they nevertheless become excited. Some men have told me that if the men engaging in a sexual encounter in the steam room are "trolls" they do not want to see it, and find it disgusting; however if the guys doing it are "hot" not only do they want to see, and do, but become interested in participating as well.

Criticism toward sexuality in the locker room is often backed up by the fact that we are no longer out-of-control teenage boys. But for many gay men, the erotic response is not really different from an adolescent one, and the line is so blurred that the argument is not well founded. Furthermore, an erection triggered by the sight of another man we find attractive is for many men, as Esteban points out, a physical reaction they still have very little control over. In fact, this was one of the reasons given to me by men who told me they prefer not to shower at the gym: they do not want to be in a situation where they are sexually excited in a place they find inappropriate for sex.

Something else that complicates this entire discussion is the level of honesty, or lack thereof, when discussing the subject. I have talked to gay men whom I have noticed cruise the locker room quite a bit and heard them complain that the locker room is too cruisy. I have noticed that even the most reserved guys at the gym casually take a peek as they walk near the shower/steam room area. This is understandable: with the reputation that some gyms have, it is difficult not to at least be curious. This curiosity is the basis for the underlying contradictions we find between truth and falacy when discussing this topic. We know what we ought to say to come across as proper and honorable, and we know how to filter our actions, reactions, and statements to please moral code. However, we often do so at the expense of suppressing our true feelings, and at times political correctness unfortunately keep us from having truly honest discussions.

Moral opinions that discourage public sexual encounters are not going to change anytime soon, but neither is our biology. The controversies regarding the sexual dynamics of the locker room will continue just as much as the debate of whether we should or should not. And for men, whether gay, bisexual, or straight, if nothing else, the issue will remain one that we will continue to be excited and conflicted about, sometimes simultaneously, as long as men continue to produce testosterone.

Notes

Chapter 2

1. Daniel Harris, *The Rise and Fall of Gay Culture* (New York: Hyperion, 1997) year), 86-110.
2. K.J. Dover, *Greek Homosexuality* (New York: Random House, 1980), 2.
3. Plato *Symposium,* 192a.
4. Thomas F. Scanlon, *Eros and Greek Athletics* (New York: Oxford University Press, 2002), 3, 8.
5. Cicero *Tusculan Disputations* 4.70.
6. David Sansone, *Greek Athletics and the Genesis of Sport* (Berkeley and Los Angeles, CA: University of California Press, 1988) 77.
7. Homer, *The Iliad,* 23.
8. Plato, *The Republic: The Complete and Unabridged Jowett Translation* (New York: Vintage Books, 1991), back cover.
9. Plato, *The Republic,* 2.376-8.
10. Plato, *Symposium,* 182 b-c.
11. Homer, *The Iliad,* 5.265-70, 20.231-5.
12. Pindar, *The Olympic Odes,* 1.44, 10.105.
13. Boswell, *Same-Sex Unions in Premodern Europe* (New York: Villard Books, 1994), 88-93.
14. Plutarch, *Life of Pelopidas,* 18.
15. E. Norman Gardiner, *Athletics of the Ancient World* (London: Oxford at the Clarendon Press, 1930), 57.
16. Ibid., 55-7.
17. Ibid., 33.
18. Kenneth R. Dutton, *The Perfectible Body, The Western Ideal of Male Physical Development* (New York: The Continuum Publishing Company, 1995), 25-6.
19. Sansone, *Greek Athletics and the Genesis of Sport,* 77.
20. Gardiner, *Athletics of the Ancient World,* 53.
21. Dover, *Greek Homosexuality,* 54-5.
22. Gardiner, *Athletics of the Ancient World,* 73-8.
23. Ibid., 73.
24. Scanlon, *Eros and Greek Athletics,* 83.
25. Ibid., 219.
26. Lactantius, *Divinae Institutions,* I.20.
27. Theognis of Megara, *Elegiae,* 2.1335-36.

Muscle Boys: Gay Gym Culture
Published by The Haworth Press, Taylor & Francis Group, 2008.
doi:10.1300/6034_13

Chapter 3

1. Plutarch *Roman Questions* 40.274.

2. Craig A. Williams, *Roman Homosexuality, Ideologies of Masculinity in Classical Antiquity* (New York: Oxford University Press, 1999), 70.

3. John Boswell, *Same-Sex Unions in Premodern Europe* (New York: Villard Books, 1994), 80.

4. Ibid., 84.

5. Ibid., 85-86.

6. Kenneth R. Dutton, *The Perfectible Body, The Western Ideal of Male Physical Development* (New York: The Continuum Publishing Company, 1995), 60.

7. David L. Chapman, *Sandow the Magnificent: Eugen Sandow and the Beginnings of Bodybuilding* (Chicago: University of Illinois Press, 1994), 3.

8. Ibid., Preface.

9. Ibid., 16-7, 33.

10. Ibid., 51.

11. Ibid.

12. Ibid., 5.

Chapter 4

1. Robert Mainardi, Interview with the author, December 2004.

2. Ibid.

3. David L. Chapman, *Sandow the Magnificent: Eugen Sandow and the Beginnings of Bodybuilding* (Chicago: University of Illinois Press, 1994), 108-9.

4. Robert Ernst, *Weakness Is a Crime: The Life of Bernarr Macfadden* (Syracuse, New York: Syracuse University Press, 1991), 17.

5. Ibid., 21.

6. Ibid., 39.

7. Ibid., 41-4.

8. Ibid., 47-9.

9. Ibid., 21-54.

10. Charles Kaiser, *The Gay Metropolis: 1940-1996* (London: Weidenfeld & Nicolson, 1998), II and III.

11. F. Valentine Hooven, III, *Beefcake: The Muscle Magazines of America 1950-1970* (Germany: Benedikt Taschen, 1995), 26-32.

12. Dennis Bell, Interview with the author, November 2004.

13. Ibid.

14. Ibid.

15. Hooven, *Beefcake: The Muscle MagazineMagazines of America 1950-1970* (Benedickt Teschen Verlag), 50.

16. Hooven, 74.

17. Harry B. Paschall, "Let Me Tell You a Fairy Tale," *Strength & Health Magazine,* June 1957, 17.

18. Robert Mainardi.

19. *Manual Enterprises v. Day,* 370 U.S. 478 (1962).

20. *Manual Entrprises v. Day,* 370 U.S. 478 (1962).

21. *Miller v. California,* 413 U.S. 15 (1973).
22. Dennis Bell, interview with the author, November 2004.
23. John Rutherford, interview with the author, October 2004.
24. Tim Adams, "Mad about the boys," *The Observer* (UK), Sunday June 30, 2002, http://observer.guardian.co.uk/review/story/0,,746475,00.html (Accessed August 25, 2005).
25. Bill Sanderson, interview with the author, November 2004.
26. Andy Wysocki, interview with the author, November 2004.
27. John Rutherford.
28. Dennis Bell.

Chapter 5

1. Michael Meehan, interview with the author, October 2004.
2. Ibid.
3. Robert Mainardi, interview with the author, December 2004.
4. Ibid.
5. Michael Meehan.
6. Anonymous.
7. Eric Friedman, interview with the author, November 2004.
8. Robert Mainardi.
9. Anonymous.

Chapter 6

1. Adam Boardman, interview with the author, October 2004.
2. Brendan Eaton, interview with the author, October 2004.
3. Tom Madonna, interview with the author, September 2004.
4. Adam Boardman.
5. Brendan Eaton.
6. Adam Boardman.
7. Ibid.
8. Brendan Eaton.
9. Ibid.
10. Ibid.
11. Ibid.
12. Adam Boardman.
13. Brendan Eaton.
14. Tom Madonna.
15. Ibid.
16. Brendan Eaton.
17. Ibid.
18. Ibid.
19. Tom Madonna.

Chapter 7

1. Lawrence K. Altman (1981). "Rare Cancer Seen in 41 Homosexuals: Outbreak Occurs Among Men in New York and California–8 Died Inside 2 Years," *New York Times,* July 3, sec. A.
2. Robert Wallace, interview with the author, July 2002.
3. Alex Cabot, interview with the author, August 2002.
4. Lawrence Price, interview with the author, July 2006.
5. Michael Mooney, interview with the author. April 2004.
6. Ibid.
7. Lennart Moller, interview with the author, December 2004.
8. Ibid.
9. Ron Tripp, interview with the author, December 2003.
10. Ibid.
11. David C. Nieman , *Fitness and Sports Medicine: An introduction* (Palo Alto, CA: Bull Publishing Company, 1990), 255.
12. Ibid.
13. Lennart Moller.
14. Ibid.
15. United States Department of Justice, Drug Enforcement Administration, "Steroid Facts," http://www.usdoj.gov/dea/concern/steroids_factsheet.html (accessed March 18, 2006).
16. U.S. Department of Health and Human Services (2000). National Institute on Drug Abuse, Research Report Series, "Steroid Abuse and Addiction." http://www.nida.nih.gov/ResearchReports/Steroids/AnabolicSteroids.html (accessed March 18, 2006).
17. Jason Six, interview with the author, October 2004.
18. Lennart Moller.

Chapter 8

1. Scott Robinson, interview with the author, August 2003.
2. Raymond Pajek, interview with the author, December 2004.
3. Ibid.
4. Scott Robinson.
5. Wayne R. Dynes (Ed.), Warren Johansson and William A. Percy (Associate Eds.), *Encyclopedia of Homosexuality* (New York and London: Garland Publishing, Inc. 1990), 555-6, 659-0.
6. Ibid.
7. Ibid., 668-9.
8. *Merriam Webster's Collegiate Dictionary,* 10th ed., S.V. "stereotype."
9. Anonymous.
10. Raymond Pajek.
11. Ibid.
12. Scott Robinson.
13. John De Cecco, interview with the author, November 2004.
14. Ibid.

15. Ibid.
16. *Team San Francisco* Newsletter, March 2001.
17. Federation of Gay Games, "Games Can Change the World" brochure (San Francisco 2001).
18. Ibid.
19. Mubarak Dahir, "Winter Games, Olympic-size closet, Where are all the out lesbian and gay athletes at the 2002 Winter Olympics in Salt Lake City?" *The Advocate,* February 19, 2002, 13.
20. David Kopay and Perry Deane Young, *The David Kopay Story: An Extraordinary Self-Revelation* (New York: Arbor House, 1977), 3, 4.
21. Glenn Burke with Erik Sherman, *Out at Home: The Glenn Burke Story* (New York: Excel Publishing 1995).
22. Dave Pallone with Alan Steinberg, *Behind the Mask: My Double Life in Baseball* (New York: Viking, 1990), 1.
23. Billy Bean with Chris Bull, *Going the Other Way: Lessons from a Life in and out of Major League Baseball* (New York: Marlowe & Company, 2003).
24. Mike Freeman, *Bloody Sundays: Inside the Dazzling, Rough-and-tumble World of the NFL* (New York: HarperCollins, 2003), p. 149.
25. Roy Simmons and Damon DiMarco, *Out of Bounds: Coming out of Sexual Abuse, Addiction, and My Life of Lies in the NFL Closet* (New York: Carroll and Graff, 2006).
26. Esera Tuaolo with John Rosengren, *Alone in the Trenches: My Life As a Gay Man in the NFL* (Illinois: Sourcebooks, Inc. 2006).
27. ESPN, http://www.espn.com (accessed September 12, 2003, no longer available).
28. John Amaechi with Chris Bull, *Man in the Middle* (New York: ESPN Books 2007).

Chapter 9

1. The Saint 1980-81, opening season membership invitation. Courtesy of boyscape.com.
2. "White Party Week Events," *Wire,* November 27, 2003, 42-45.
3. John Putnam, interview with the author, July 2005.
4. Ibid.
5. Ibid.
6. Scott Cullens, interview with the author, July 2003.
7. Ibid.
8. Corey Jennings.
9. Ibid.
10. Ibid.
11. Corey Jennings.
12. Ibid.
13. Anonymous.
14. John Putnam.
15. Corey Jennings.

16. Scott Cullens.
17. Ibid.

Chapter 10

1. Gary Phoenix, interview with the author, December 2004.
2. Paul Flynn, "Is the potbelly the new gay ideal?" *The Guardian* (UK), April 18, 2003. http://www.guardian.co.uk/style/story/0,,939097,00.html (accessed March 27, 2006).
3. Andrew Sullivan, *Salon.com,* August 1, 2003. http://archive.salon.com/opinion/sullivan/2003/08/01/bears/index.html (accessed August 1, 2003, no longer available).
4. Cynthia Laird, "Bears Rendezvous in SF this weekend," *Bay Area Reporter,* 13 February 2003, 12.
5. Luke Cottrill, interview with the author, August 2003.
6. Ibid.
7. *Bear Magazine,* July 1998, cover.
8. Gary Phoenix.
9. Ibid.
10. Jay DeMarco, interview with the author, August 2003.
11. Luke Cottrill.
12. Anonymous.
13. Anonymous.
14. Jay DeMarco.
15. Gary Phoenix.
16. Luke Cottrill.
17. Jay DeMarco.
18. Luke Cottrill.

Chapter 11

1. Leonard Simpson, interview with the author, December 2003.
2. Michael Meehan, interview with the author, October 2004.
3. John Amodio, interview with the author, November 2004.
4. Leonard Simpson.
5. American College of Sports Medicine, *Resource Manual for Guidelines for Exercise Testing and Prescription,* Second Edition (Philadelphia: Lea & Febiger, 1993), 571.
6. Leonard Simpson.
7. President's Council on Physical Fitness and Sports, Research Digest (March 2002), "Cost and Consequences of Sedentary Living: New Battleground for an Old Enemy." http://www.fitness.gov/researchdigestmarch2002.pdf (accessed August 24, 2007).
8. Cecil Franco, interview with the author, October 2004.
9. Ibid.
10. Ibid.
11. Lennart Moller, interview with the author, December 2004.

12. Ibid.

13. Nancy Etcoff, *Survival of the Prettiest: The Science of Beauty* (New York: Anchor Books, 2000), 24.

14. John Amodio.

15. Leonard Simpson.

16. Michelangelo Signorile, *Life Outside: The Signorile Report on Gay Men: Sex, Drugs, Muscles, and the Passages of Life* (New York: HarperCollins, 1997), 266-293.

17. Cecil Franco.

18. Brian Heaphy, "The Social and Policy Implications of Non-Heterosexual Aging" (Study conducted with Andrew Yip and Debbie Thompson at Nottingham Trent University), 2003. http://www.esrcsocietytoday.ac.uk/ESRCInfoCentre/PO/releases/2003/september/growingold.aspx?ComponentId=2175&SourcePageId=1404 (accessed March 28, 2006).

19. John Amodio.

20. Leonard Simpson.

21. Cecil Franco.

22. Michael Meehan.

23. Leonard Simpson.

Chapter 12

1. Esteban Soto, interview with the author, November 2004.
2. Cecil Franco, interview with the author, November 2004.
3. Ibid.
4. Esteban Soto.
5. *Lawrence et al. v. Texas,* 539 U.S. 558 (2003).
6. Jason Six, interview with the author, October 2004.
7. Tom Madonna, interview with the author, September 2004.
8. Jason Six.
9. Damon Xiang, interview with the author, September 2004.
10. Jason Six.

Index

Page numbers followed by the letter "i" indicate illustrations.

Muscle Boys: Gay Gym Culture
Published by The Haworth Press, Taylor & Francis Group, 2008.

doi:10.1300/6034_14

For Product Safety Concerns and Information please contact our EU representative GPSR@taylorandfrancis.com
Taylor & Francis Verlag GmbH, Kaufingerstraße 24, 80331 München, Germany

www.ingramcontent.com/pod-product-compliance
Lightning Source LLC
Chambersburg PA
CBHW072050020426
42334CB00017B/1459

* 9 7 8 1 5 6 0 2 3 4 0 4 3 *